You Can Have a Better Period

A Practical Guide to Calmer and Less Painful Periods

Le'Nise Brothers

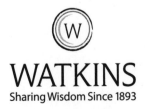

WATKINS

Sharing Wisdom Since 1893

To Mummy,

Here's the book I wish you had.

You Can Have a Better Period
Le'Nise Brothers

First published in the UK and USA in 2022 by
Watkins, an imprint of Watkins Media Limited
Unit 11, Shepperton House, 83–93 Shepperton Road
London N1 3DF

enquiries@watkinspublishing.com

Commissioning Editor: Anya Hayes
Assistant Editor: Brittany Willis
Head of Design: Karen Smith
Designer: Steve Williamson
Illustrator: Sneha Alexander
Production: Uzma Taj

A CIP record for this book is available from the British Library

ISBN: 978-1-78678-560-2

10 9 8 7 6 5 4 3 2 1

Printed in United Kingdom by TJ Books

www.watkinspublishing.com

Contents

Introduction

We all have that one friend. Her periods come like clockwork every month, with no pain and no drama. She gets on with her life and her period comes along on the ride with her. I used to think this woman had won the health lottery – she was one of the lucky ones.

You can be one of these women. You can have a period that is pain- and drama-free. You can have a menstrual cycle that syncs with the rest of your life. I promise you this isn't a fantasy!

According to the NHS, the average woman has two to three days of pain either right before her period or when she has her period.[1] That's the equivalent of between 24 and 36 days of pain each year! If this was any other condition, it's hard to believe that we would allow this to persist. Unfortunately, the inevitability of period pain has been normalized in our culture – by the way periods and menstrual health are discussed in films, magazines and on TV (usually as a huge inconvenience or trauma), by the stories that are passed on by those in our lives who have periods and, for many of us, how our mothers and sisters experienced their periods.

We now have the opportunity to change this narrative and change the way we experience and talk about our periods. Pain is a sign from our bodies that something isn't right. It's an opportunity to ask questions and dig deeper, rather than simply accepting this as part of your experience of having a period. Asking questions helps empower us to better navigate our bodies and our health.

I know so many of us have been told that it's normal to have painful periods, normal to feel like your hormones are running the show, normal to be an emotional mess before your period. I'm here to tell you that it doesn't have to be this way. This book is your guide to having a better period and understanding your menstrual cycle.

My Story

When I first thought about the book I wanted to write about periods, hormones and menstrual health, I pictured the book I wished I'd had to guide me when I was at the worst of my period problems.

My period started when I was 13. I was a late bloomer in so many ways, including being the last of my friends to get my period. When it arrived, it felt like a big moment. I was finally transitioning into the next part of my life! And it was indeed a big moment. That first period ushered in years of pain, physical and emotional distress and the start of the ongoing fight I still have with my body.

My very first period was strange because I had been waiting for it for so long. When it finally came, I was really disorientated. This new thing had moved all of my anchor points and I needed to figure out how to navigate my body in a different way.

I remember being in the bathroom, seeing the blood in the toilet and calling out to my family in the living room to say that something had happened. To which my father said, "Oh, did you get your period?" to which I replied, "Yeah, I think I did."

It was from that point onward that my body began to feel like such an unwieldy mystery to me. I started to get boobs, hips and a butt. My clothes fitted differently. I felt more and more awkward. And every month, I had to figure out how to get through this incredibly dramatic event that seemed to be affecting only me so badly. From the outside, my friends looked like they didn't have a care in the world when it came to their periods.

Don't get me wrong, I did have carefree teenage moments. I would have about three weeks when my life seemed completely normal. I could function like a normal teenager: going to school, hanging out with my friends, reading, listening to music, playing sport and having massive crushes on boys. Then I would feel the whispers of my period coming and I'd know that all hell was about to break loose. The fury and the tears would begin, then five days of terrible cramps, headaches and intensely heavy bleeding.

My attitude toward my period transformed from something I was really looking forward to into a monthly source of dread. From the very beginning, I had terribly painful and heavy periods that left me lying on the bathroom floor writhing in pain and missing days of school. The only things that seemed to resolve it were hot baths that I would sit in for hours, strong painkillers and sleep. You may be wondering: where was my mother while all this was happening?

She was trying to cope with her own period problems. For years, she had periods that seemed endless, sometimes lasting for a month at a time. She told me much later that she didn't know how she got through them, but she thought it was normal. Eventually, she was diagnosed with fibroids (non-cancerous growths on, in and within the muscular walls of the uterus) and had two removed that were the size of grapefruits. These two fibroids caused years of heavy, month-long periods that left her drained and struggling to cope. Seeing what my mother was going through made me think that having problematic periods was just a part of being a woman, something you just had to cope with.

I think back to a particular moment when I was 15 years old, laid out on my bathroom floor in agony from period pain. This was a particular type of pain that felt as though it was stabbing me all over my stomach and legs. I missed school that day and did what became a habit: running and rerunning hot baths that I would sit in for hours to try and soothe the pain. Eventually, I told my mother about my painful and heavy periods. It took some convincing (the distrust of allopathic medicine runs deep in my family!), but in time, she took me to the doctor, who told me what was happening to me was just part of having a period. She gave me a prescription for Naproxen (a strong painkiller) and birth control pills and sent me on my way.

Those pills dealt with the pain, but they did nothing for the heavy bleeding and blood clots, so I became an expert in using a combination of pads, rolled-up toilet paper and tampons to manage the flow. I can't tell you the number of underwear and trousers I bled through.

I soldiered on because I believed what the doctor told me and what I saw happening to my mother: that this was just part of being a woman. It was my lot to have painful, heavy periods, wear double pads and feel lousy for one week of every month.

How I would have loved to read a book that told me that what I was experiencing wasn't normal. That having a period didn't automatically sign me up for nearly 40 years of pain and suffering. That it wasn't my lot as a woman.

I didn't have this book – so instead, I suffered for a long time.

I hated my body for betraying me. I hated fighting with my body every time I got my period.

As I got older, I started to realize that it didn't have to be this way. Only in the last seven to eight years have I had periods that have been consistently straightforward. And for me, that's life-changing. How did I do it? Through nothing that revolutionary or dramatic: eating loads of vegetables, not drinking alcohol, not eating a lot of sugar or dairy, managing my stress (and being really clear about my boundaries), having a consistent yoga practice, deep breathing and great sleep. When something changes (like living through a pandemic and all of the changes this has brought!), I know exactly what to do to get back to a better place. And that's what I want for you.

Helping You Have a Better Period

When you picked this book up, did you scoff a little at the title? Did you think, "There's no way I can have a better period"? If that's you, I'd like to encourage you to put aside your reservations and read this book with an open mind.

This book for is anyone who has a period: women, non-binary folk and transgender men. For brevity, I do use the terms woman, women and female throughout the book. The best way to read this is straight through. However, you're more than welcome to flip forward to the chapters on each phase of the menstrual cycle and start at whichever phase you're currently in. If you're thinking, "Whoa, Le'Nise, I didn't even know that the menstrual cycle had different phases!", don't worry, I've got you. We'll dive into that in Part 2.

I want you to know that you don't have to live with period pain, heavy bleeding or an emotional rollercoaster. That's not an inevitable part of having a period. In my private nutrition practice, I see and speak to women from all walks of life, and two things are clear: period problems don't discriminate, and women continue to believe pain and suffering are a normal part of having a period.

What if I told you they aren't? What if I told you that it's possible to have a period that just happens every menstrual cycle and is as commonplace as changing your underwear every day? Something you do without comment or drama. I believe that once we change our understanding of what's normal and what isn't (painful and heavy periods aren't normal!), we change our view of what's going on in our bodies and what we're willing to live with.

5

My own period story has a happier ending. Little by little, I stopped taking the birth control pill, started to make small changes to what I ate, how I exercised and how I managed my stress. Gradually, I started to see improvements in the quality of my period each menstrual cycle. It became less painful, lighter and less dramatic.

My period isn't perfect. I know that if I eat a lot of sugary foods one month (this definitely happened during the first Covid lockdown!), I will see the effects of this in my next menstrual cycle. But I'm okay with this, because first, I need to live my life and, second, I know this pain is temporary and I have the tools to fix it.

Are you ready to make the changes that can help you have better periods?

My hope is that this book gives you the tools to help you tune into your body – so you know what's normal for you – and then change your menstrual health for the better. I want to help educate you on why periods are important, so that you understand why the nutrition and lifestyle changes I'll be taking you through in this book will make a difference for the long term.

We'll talk about the menstrual cycle and why this is our fifth vital sign. I'll talk through the power of the female body and what we gain from harnessing the different physical, emotional and mental strengths that occur during each of the four phases of our menstrual cycle. For example, you'll learn why your libido might be stronger during certain times of your menstrual cycle. You'll also learn what hormones actually are, how they guide us, why we're all a bit hormonal and what makes that a good thing!

Learning what's normal and what isn't will change your expectations of your body and yourself. In Part 2, we'll go through actions you can take during each phase of your menstrual cycle to improve your physical, menstrual and emotional health. In each chapter, I share specific nutrition, exercise and lifestyle recommendations for each phase that you can come back to again and again. We'll also look at painful periods, mood changes and missing or irregular periods in detail in Chapters 8, 9 and 10.

Finally, we'll look at how we can put the entire menstrual cycle together so that we can begin to spot patterns and see the effects of changes to the way we eat, move and in our lifestyle choices.

My goal for this book is to give you the tools I use in my private practice as a nutritionist to help you have a better period. My own journey to heal my period and overall health inspired me to leave a 15-year career in advertising and retrain as a nutritionist, eventually specializing in women's health, hormones and the menstrual cycle.

After reading this book, I'd love for you to understand the power of our natural feminine rhythm and cycle, so that you feel that you are in control of, rather than held captive by, your period and menstrual cycle. I'm tired of women feeling that pain and emotional drama are a normal part of having a period. I'm tired of women planning their lives around heavy and painful periods and feeling like they're missing out. I'm tired of women believing the myth that period pain is normal.

I wrote this book because I want you to have a better period.

PART 1

Changing Expectations

CHAPTER 1
Are Periods Supposed to Be Painful?

Let's go all the way back to the beginning. How did you first learn about your period and menstrual cycle? At school? From a parent, friend or family member? Did you have to figure it out on your own? My own menstrual health education was pretty scant. I remember a class when I was 12 where we learned the basics: how to use tampons and pads, to expect to bleed each month, to ask our parents for painkillers if the pain got too strong. That was it. I'm going pretty far back into the recesses of my memory here, but I don't recall an extensive menstrual education at school. We spent more time talking about how to avoid getting pregnant than learning about the impact that our periods and hormones would have on the next 35 to 40 years of our lives, which is so wild when you consider just how many periods we have over that many years.

It was only once my husband and I decided to start trying to conceive a child that I started to educate myself. I began reading everything I could get my hands on, learning about ovulation, the importance of cervical fluid, the changes in my hormones and neurotransmitters during my menstrual cycle and how what I ate and drank could make a difference. It was eye-opening, to say the least. Over and over, I kept thinking: "I wish I had learned this earlier." I had spent years living with tough period pain and heavy periods, from what I know is likely to be mild endometriosis. This knowledge could have been life-changing.

Celebrating Our Periods

Cultural stories, religious beliefs and taboos play a huge role in what we think, and how we learn about, our periods. They influence why so many of us don't know much about our periods, don't understand our menstrual cycle, or simply believe that putting up with pain, a heavy flow or emotional turmoil is a normal part of having a period.

Even today, menstrual stigma continues. Think about the times you might have slipped a tampon up your sleeve or hidden your menstrual products in a special bag before going to the washroom. In a survey commissioned as part of their #NoShameHere campaign, the period equity charity Bloody Good Period found that 97 per cent of respondents had hidden period products because it's the norm, 76 per cent had hidden period products because of embarrassment and 56 per cent had hidden period products because of shame.[1]

Where does this shame and embarrassment come from? My belief is that there are both cultural and religious roots to menstrual stigma. Most religions refer to menstruating women as ritually unclean. Think of the adverts that use blue fluid to depict menstrual blood. Think of the taboo around period sex (actually a fantastic time to have sex because orgasms can reduce menstrual cramps!) or the furtive way many of us first learned about periods or spoke about them with friends. These touchpoints begin to help us understand why menstruation is thought of as dirty or something to be hidden. When you layer on a cultural belief that menstruation leads women to be physically or mentally disordered,[2] we can start to understand why the unfortunate stigma around menstruation persists.

In Orthodox Judaism, the Torah calls women who are menstruating and haven't had a purity bath *niddah* and enforces strict separation between a menstruating woman and her husband. The book of Leviticus, one of the five books of the Torah, states: "When a woman has a discharge, her discharge being blood from her body, she shall remain in her impurity for seven days; whoever touches her shall be unclean until evening ... and if any man lies with her at all and her blood be upon him, he will be unclean for seven days." At the end of her period, the woman is responsible for going to the *mikveh*, a Jewish ritual bath, where she will become clean. Beyond the focus on cleanliness, there is something special about having a ritual to mark the end of your period. Interestingly, some Jewish feminists have embraced *niddah* as a time of spiritual renewal, akin to what I call going into the period cave. They have also reframed the *mikveh* as a place devoted to celebrating female biological function.[3]

By way of contrast, Guru Nanak, the founder of Sikhism, openly chides those who say menstruating women are spiritually polluted, saying that a mother's blood is necessary for human life and therefore sacred.[4]

In Nepal, culture and religion intersect, especially for those living in rural areas. The ancient Hindu practice of *chhaupadi*, meaning "untouchable being", prohibits Hindu women and girls from participating in normal family activities while menstruating, as they are considered impure and unclean. Although the Nepalese government made this practice illegal in 2018, it persists in rural Nepal,[5] where menstruating women are isolated in poorly ventilated *chhau* huts, livestock sheds or courtyards outside their home.[6] They are unable to visit temples, use other villagers' kitchen utensils or wash in communal water sources. As recently as 2019, a woman and her two children died from suffocation after she barricaded them into a windowless menstrual hut during her period.[7] Even in wider Nepalese society, the beliefs that menstruation is spiritually polluting and taboo persist.[8]

Let's consider why the belief that periods are supposed to be painful and messy endures. Research has shown that knowledge gaps or deficits in knowledge create confusion as to whether the cultural restrictions and taboos being passed down about menstruation are actually accurate.[9] My own Afro-Caribbean background comes to mind here. The belief that painful periods are inevitable had been passed down without question throughout the generations of religious women in my family. In hushed conversations, we learned we needed to endure when facing pain. These beliefs perhaps had roots in the Biblical verse of Genesis 3:16: "To the woman he said, 'I will make your pains in childbearing very severe; with painful labour you will give birth to children.'"[10] This was corroborated by what we saw in the lived experience of our female family members. As you read in the introduction to this book, I saw my mother's pain and suffering and expected the same. Throughout this book, I encourage you to question whether cultural and religious beliefs have given you a negative attitude toward menstruation. If the answer is yes, could you ask yourself if there's room to change your beliefs?

Is it possible to have a more positive view of menstruation, or even to celebrate it? Let's look at cultures both past and present.

In ancient Rome and Greece, menstruating women were seen as extraordinarily powerful. According to Pliny the Elder, the Roman author and philosopher, "A menstruating woman who uncovers her body can scare away hailstorms, whirlwinds, and lightning. If she strips naked and walks around the field, caterpillars, worms and beetles fall off the ears of corn."[11] I don't think I'll be walking through central London naked in a thunderstorm any time soon, but it's nice to know that the immense, fiery power of menstruating women was acknowledged at one time.

In the present day, the Apaches, a Native American tribe, hold a four-day Sunrise Dance, which is an elaborate series of rituals that begin at menarche (the onset of the first period) and prepares girls for the transition into puberty. In Apache, this is called *Isánáklésh Gotal*, a term which encompasses the process by which the girl is transformed into the Apache heroine Isánáklésh. It is believed that through her participation in the rigours and demands of the Sunrise Dance and the extended puberty rites, including a series of physical and mental tests that continue for several months afterwards, the girl gains a greater sense of her identity and purpose in the Apache tribe.[12]

In contrast to the tradition of *chhaupadi* described earlier, some Hindus in India believe that menstruation, especially the first menstrual period, is an occasion worth marking. South Indian families hold a coming-of-age ceremony called *ritusuddhi* or *Ritu Kala Samskara*, in which the girl wears a traditional outfit called a *langa voni,* or a half sari, and receives presents, including her first full or half sari.[13] This can be a complex event lasting up to 16 days.

On my podcast, *Period Story*, I've had conversations with a few women whose parents and family made a big deal of their first periods, using it as an occasion to mark the transition from girlhood to young womanhood.

One of my guests, Tamu Thomas, talked about the mixed feelings she had about the excitement this rite of passage caused in her family. Before her first period arrived, she'd been really excited. Once it arrived, Tamu recalls: "There was all this hoopla about me joining the club that I didn't want. My mum bought me this kit, it was bright fuchsia pink and it had tampons and sanitary towels." Tamu was excited about having her first period, but this was eclipsed by having it shared by her entire family. As an adult she now understands, "It's a big coming-of-age thing, it's a huge marker in human development, in female development, and my mum was celebrating that. But I thought a period was just for me and no one else to know about and I carried that belief with me for a very long time."

I wonder how we would feel if our first periods were celebrated joyously rather than hidden away in shame and silence. How would we feel if we knew that our menstrual cycle could be a positive force in our lives to be harnessed for its power, rather than something to dread?

Having a better understanding of menstruation, hormone health and how our bodies work is the first step toward removing the stigma. When we talk about what's normal and what it isn't, we can develop positive attitudes about our periods and challenge negative assumptions.

This enables us to push back against culturally accepted norms about periods. Think about these questions:

- Do you think period pain is normal because that's all you've ever experienced?
- Do you think heavy periods are normal because of what you've heard from friends and family?
- Do you accept pain, a heavy bleed and mood changes because your doctor has told you it's normal?

Have you ever gently questioned the origin of your beliefs about your period? As you read through this book, notice if your attitudes begin to change.

In this book, we'll go back to basics, starting with understanding that our menstrual cycle and period are one of our five vital signs. We'll move through each phase, so we understand what's happening to our bodies during our periods and the rest of our menstrual cycle. You'll also find practical support for period problems and beyond in the later chapters of the book. We'll explore nutrition and lifestyle supports for reducing and managing period pain, missing and irregular periods, heavy periods and the other menstrual symptoms (including PMS!) that we've been told are a normal part of having a period. Let's get into it!

CHAPTER 2
Why Your Menstrual Cycle Is Your Fifth Vital Sign

What does the word vital mean to you? Essential? Fundamental? Something you can't live without? When it comes to our health, we have a small group of important signals from the body that tell us how the most critical parts of our health are functioning. These are our vital signs. When you go to the doctor or hospital, they will check your pulse or heart rate, body temperature, breath or respiration rate and blood pressure to get a basic understanding of your current health status. Would it surprise you to learn that your menstrual cycle is another key indicator of your overall health?

As you read this book, you'll learn why our entire menstrual cycle, including our period and ovulation, must be considered another vital sign. Here's another way to look at it: if you don't have a period and you're not pregnant, you get worried, don't you? A delayed period is a sign that something's off. If you don't ovulate every menstrual cycle and you're not on hormonal contraception, it's a sign that you need to investigate further. You might be thinking, "My period is so awful, I would be happy for it to disappear!" I can relate. When my period was at its worst, I spent a lot of time wishing it away. My hope is that as you read this book, you'll add different foods, supplements and practices that begin a positive shift toward improving your period over time. At the least, I'd love it if you thought slightly differently about your menstrual health.

The American College of Obstetricians and Gynecologists recommends the inclusion of the menstrual cycle as one of our vital signs,[1] deeming it just as important as the others for evaluating overall health status. Unfortunately, in the UK, the NHS don't yet have a similar view on the importance of the menstrual cycle, but I hope this will change soon.

If the menstrual cycle is so critical, why don't we learn more about it in school? That's a great question. As I explained in the introduction, I only learned about my menstrual cycle, beyond my period, when I was trying to have a child. This seems to be a common experience, but this is changing. Menstrual health education was made compulsory in schools in England in 2020 and there are campaigns for this to be extended to the rest of the UK.

When I began this project, I scribbled this on a Post-it note and pinned it above my desk: "Write the book you would have wanted to read when you got your period." As I've been writing, my eyes keep flicking back to this note, helping focus my mind (and words!) on helping you understand the value and importance of your menstrual health.

This is where we come back to the significance of treating our menstrual cycle like a vital sign. When something is off, it's a message from our body, and we need to stop ignoring these messages or treating them like they're supposed to be there. Pain is a common example of this. We treat period pain like it's a normal response from the body. Many of us learn this from those around us, and even from medical professionals: it's just a part of having a period and we should accept it. As I explain in more detail in Chapters 4 and 8, we just wouldn't accept this with any other condition. We wouldn't tell someone with tooth pain to just deal with it, would we? We'd tell them to phone their dentist and get it sorted. This is why treating our periods, ovulation and menstrual cycle like a vital sign empowers us to seek help and support. We know what's normal, what isn't, and we can act accordingly.

To truly see our menstrual cycle as a vital sign, we need to understand every part of it. We'll go into the details of each phase in this book, but it's helpful to start with a basic overview, especially if some of this information is new to you.

The Four Phases of the Menstrual Cycle

Our periods are what we tend to focus on when we think about our menstrual cycles. This is mostly due to the negative experiences many of us have had with our bleeds, including painful periods and mood changes, which I explore in Chapters 8 and 9. Let's zoom out and look beyond our periods to our menstrual cycles as a whole.

There are four phases of the menstrual cycle: menstruation, follicular, ovulatory and luteal. The length of each phase will vary depending on the individual, but we would roughly expect the overall menstrual cycle to last between 21 and 35 days. You may have learned that our menstrual cycle should be 28 days; however, many of us have cycles that are shorter or longer and vary by a few days each time. This is normal.

In writing this chapter, I got curious about my own cycle and looked back on the data from my period tracker. I have almost eight years of information! As I scrolled back, I could see that my cycles have been between 22 and 26 days long for the last eight years. I thought this was abnormal for a long time and I wondered what was wrong with me. Why didn't I have 28-day menstrual cycles? It's only since educating myself that I understand that I have nothing to worry about. I know that my cycle is highly sensitive to stress and if I have a few months when I'm more stressed than usual, my cycles will veer toward 22 or 23 days.

A quick note: your menstrual cycle is not the same as your period. I've heard some women refer to their period as their cycle, which has resulted in some confusion when I start talking about the menstrual cycle and how long we should expect it to be!

The Four Phases

Phase	Inner Season	Keywords	Approximate Number of Days
Menstruation	Winter	Surrender, rest, reflect	3–7
Follicular	Spring	Play, energize, begin	6–11
Ovulatory	Summer	Celebrate, dare, connect	5
Luteal	Autumn	Slow down, organize, breathe	10–14

I love the analogy of the phases of the menstrual cycle as seasons. This was originated by the founders of the Red School, Alexandra Pope and Sjanie Hugo Wurlitzer. In their 2017 book *Wild Power*, they say that throughout your menstrual month, you move through an inner winter, spring, summer, autumn and back again. Each phase brings a set of specific resources and psychological challenges that help you grow into yourself and your power. My friend Jen Wright, the founder of menstrual- and lunar-cycle journal company Life, Aligned, compiled the keywords in the table above to guide each season. This is such a fantastic way of thinking about our menstrual cycle because it shifts it away from being a negative experience focused on menstruation to something that reflects the ongoing cyclical changes we experience. It means that if menstruation is hard for you (right now!), you know that you have the beautiful time of your inner spring and summer to look forward to.

I find it helpful to split the menstrual cycle into four phases, because there is so much happening during each phase. However, most medical practitioners tend to split the menstrual cycle into two parts: follicular (focusing on procreation and conception) and luteal (focusing on getting ready for menstruation), with ovulation sitting in the middle. It's worth bearing this in mind if your doctor or healthcare practitioner isn't familiar with the four phases of the menstrual cycle.

We'll do a deep dive into each of the four phases so that you understand the changes to your hormonal, energetic, nutrition and exercise needs and even your mental and emotional state. You'll understand why you feel so confident and more willing to take risks during one phase and more risk-averse and inwardly focused in another. And this has benefits beyond your physical health. It can even make you work and study differently and change your expectations for your personal relationships.

Hormones and Neurotransmitters

Do any of the following phrases seem familiar to you?

- "My hormones are controlling me!"
- "I'm so hormonal!"
- "My hormones are driving me crazy!"

It seems to me that we've positioned hormones as bad, and we blame them for the less positive parts of our menstrual cycle. I'd like to change that. We have over 50 different hormones covering different bodily functions including hydration, growth, energy, hunger, healing, blood pressure, blood sugar and metabolism, stress response and reproduction.

With hormones and neurotransmitters, I prefer to think of them as guiding, rather than controlling, our bodily functions, almost akin to the way an orchestra works together to play a beautiful piece of music.

Let's make an important distinction between hormones and neurotransmitters before we go any further.

Hormones: chemical messengers that move through the bloodstream and send messages to hormone receptors on different parts of our body. For example, oestrogen is a hormone primarily produced by the ovaries, with receptors on our bone, brain and skin cells (and more). They use a lock-and-key function: the hormone is the key and the hormone receptor is the lock.

Neurotransmitters: chemical messengers used by the nervous system to communicate signals from nerve cells to receptors on cells in the muscles, glands and other nerves. For example, acetylcholine, a neurotransmitter important for learning and memory, will attach to acetylcholine receptors in the brain, muscles and heart.

Some chemicals act as both a hormone and a neurotransmitter and so you will find them in both tables on the next few pages. One example of this is serotonin.

When it comes to menstrual health, we usually only hear about oestrogen and progesterone. Behind the scenes, there are a wide range of hormones and neurotransmitters that rise and fall during each phase of our menstrual cycle. As you read through each chapter, you'll learn about these fascinating chemicals. The tables below include the most relevant hormones and neurotransmitters to menstrual health. You can refer back to them as you read, if you need clarification.

My hope is that the more you understand about how hormones and neurotransmitters affect our menstrual health, you'll better understand your body and perhaps change your expectations about what you can and can't do. As we'll explore in the next section, our cyclical nature brings certain strengths to the forefront during different phases of our menstrual cycle.

Hormones

Category	Hormones	Where It's Produced	Role
Reproduction	Oestrogen (oestradiol, oestrone, oestriol, oestetrol)	Ovaries, adrenal glands, adipose tissue, fetus, placenta	Feminizing hormone, has many functions, including growth of uterine lining and bone, cardiovascular and skin health
	Progesterone	Ovaries	Produced after ovulation, calming and anti-inflammatory, many other functions
	Testosterone	Adrenal glands, ovaries	Supports muscle growth, bone density, libido
	Follicle Stimulating Hormone (FSH)	Pituitary gland	Stimulates maturation of Graafian follicles
	Luteinizing Hormone (LH)	Pituitary gland	Signals release of the mature egg from ovary
	Gonadotropin-releasing Hormone (GnRH)	Hypo-thalamus	Signals the release of FSH and LH from the pituitary gland
	Dehydroepi-androsterone (DHEA)	Adrenal glands, ovaries	Helps make oestrogen and testosterone
	Androstenedione	Adrenal glands, ovaries	Helps make oestrogen and testosterone
	Prolactin	Pituitary gland	Promotes milk production in the breasts
	Pregnenolone	Adrenal glands	Helps make oestrogen, testosterone, cortisol, progesterone
Energy and Hunger	Leptin	Adipose tissue	Signals fullness and satiety
	Ghrelin	Stomach	Stimulates appetite and hunger
	Insulin	Pancreas	Helps bring sugar into cells
	Cholecystokinin (CCK)	Duodenum	Releases digestive enzymes from pancreas and bile from gallbladder

Category	Hormones	Where It's Produced	Role
Stress	Adrenaline	Adrenal glands	Manages the body's stress response, i.e. fight or flight
	Noradrenaline	Adrenal glands	Manages the body's stress response, i.e. fight or flight
	Cortisol	Adrenal glands	Manages the body's stress response, affects metabolism and immune system
	Corticotropin-releasing Hormone (CRH)	Hypo-thalamus	Central driver of stress response system, cause releases of ACTH
	Adrenocortico-tropic Hormone (ACTH)	Pituitary gland	Causes secretion of cortisol
Temperature and Metabolism	Thyrotropin-releasing Hormone (TRH)	Hypo-thalamus	Controls the release of TSH and prolactin
	Thyroid-stimulating Hormone (TSH)	Pituitary gland	Controls the production and release of T4 and T3
	Thyroxine (T4)	Thyroid gland	Inactive thyroid hormone, converted to T3 to regulate body temperature, digestion and reproduction
	Triiodothyronine (T3)	Thyroid gland	Active thyroid hormone, works with T4 to regulate body temperature, digestion and reproduction
	Parathyroid Hormone (PTH)	Parathyroid gland	Regulates calcium levels in the blood
	Vitamin D	Kidneys	Supports bone health, is required to absorb calcium from the gut to the bloodstream
Mood and Sleep	Oxytocin	Hypo-thalamus	Contracts the uterus during childbirth, promotes lactation, promotes trust and recognition
	Melatonin	Digestive tract, brain, pineal gland	Helps us go to sleep and stay asleep
	Serotonin	Digestive tract, brain	Supports appetite, digestion and bowel function

Neurotransmitters

Category	Neurotransmitters	Role
Memory, Cognition, Learning	Dopamine	Connected with reward and pleasure, learning, memory and coordination
	Acetylcholine	Important for brain function and memory
	Glutamate	Has an excitatory effect on the brain, important for memory, learning
Mood	Serotonin	Helps regulate mood, sleep and our body clock
	Endorphins	Inhibit pain signals and give us the feel-good factor
	Gamma-aminobutyric acid (GABA)	Has an inhibitory action on the nervous system, calming
	Adrenaline	Manages the body's stress response
	Noradrenaline	Manages the body's stress response

What to Expect During Each Phase

The physical, biological, hormonal and mental changes we experience during each phase of our menstrual cycle are a compass we can use to guide us. We tend to have the expectation that we should feel the same, every day. When we acknowledge changing physical and mental energy, changes in mood and mental focus, we have the amazing ability to play to our strengths. It allows us to let go of any guilt for not being on 24/7.

I remember a conversation I had with a client, whom I'll call Maria. Maria was frustrated that she couldn't grind on her business goals with the same energy all month long. She worked hard and saw her period and the lack of energy she felt during this time as a betrayal. I encouraged her to begin to reframe how she looked at her period, considering it an opportunity to create space to recharge so that she could jump back into her work life feeling more energized and better than ever. We looked at how cyclical changes in hormones and neurotransmitters alter our cognitive skills, memory, mood, communication skills and mental focus. I suggested she use the introspective mental energy of the menstrual phase to focus on reviewing what was and wasn't working in her business and make big decisions. She was resistant because she had been working in 24-hour cycles for so long. Slowly but surely, being mindful of where she was in her menstrual cycle and how she was feeling helped her understand that she couldn't work the same way all cycle long, but she could work in a way that acknowledged the cyclical shifts in her mental focus.

This applies equally to our physical energy. As we'll explore, our physical energy rises and falls across our menstrual cycle, which has implications for the way you move your body, the exercise you do and even what you eat. Being aware of this helps you let go of any guilt about not being able to crush your spin class or your run every time, especially as you move to the end of your cycle toward your next period.

Phase / Inner Season	Physical Energy	Mood	Mental Focus
Menstruation / Winter	Energy at its lowest point	Reflective and inward-looking	Review and evaluation, introspection, decision-making, focus on self-care practices
Follicular / Spring	Energy starting to rise	Positive, social, outgoing, adventurous	Increased creativity and interest in starting something new
Ovulatory / Summer	Peak energy	Daring, risk-taking	Peak resilience, communication skills and confidence are at their strongest
Luteal / Autumn	Energy starting to decline	Focused, changing	Focus on what you know, getting through your to-do list, detail-orientated

Do you relate to any of this? Think back to your last period. Did you push yourself more than you needed to? Did you feel guilty about going a bit slower at work? Take some time to think about how you might do things a little differently next time.

Now that we know that our menstrual cycle is one of our five vital signs, I encourage you to explore what this means for your menstrual health experience. What is your cycle telling you? What have you been ignoring? If you're not sure yet, not to worry. In the next chapter, we'll look at what a normal menstrual cycle should look like. I hope this will continue to shift your understanding of what's happening to you. Then, in Part 2, we'll get into what you can do to begin to change things.

CHAPTER 3
What's a Normal Period and Menstrual Cycle?

I want to start this chapter by exploring the word "normal", because I know it can be a loaded term. When we say that something is normal, there is an implication that there is a standard that we should look to achieve and that anything outside of this is abnormal. There are many wonderful examples of how people are pushing back against the word normal. Take Unilever – the manufacturer of Dove, Simple and Lynx – removing the word normal from its beauty products. This is a positive step that reminds us of the diversity of our world and reflects changing beauty standards.

In the health and wellbeing space, we see similar changes. We're seeing movement away from using outdated and racist tools such as body mass index (BMI) as a marker of what is "normal" in terms of overall health. This body-measurement tool was introduced in the 19th century by the Belgian mathematician Adolphe Quetelet. His work centred around identifying the characteristics of *l'homme moyen* – "the average man" – collecting his data from white French and Scottish men. He developed the Quetelet Index to assess weight across a population, rather than on an individual basis.[1] In the 1970s, the researcher Ancel Keys popularized the use of this flawed tool as an easy means of measuring body fat, using his influence in the American medical community to push for the use of BMI over the ideal weight-to-height ratio tables used by the insurance industry,[2] eventually being used worldwide as a proxy to assess adiposity and overweight-related issues.[3]

I feel hopeful about the body positivity movement, which looks to redress body size norms, asking us to consider why white European female bodies have been seen as the standard for so long. I personally prefer body neutrality as a way of thinking of my body. For me, this means that thoughts of clothing size or weight become less important and there is an acknowledgement that some days we may feel great about ourselves and other days we might not. It doesn't mean that we hate ourselves, it simply means that we are cyclical beings with changing hormones and perspectives. Layering in the menstrual cycle here, if we think about our inner spring and summer, we're more likely to feel more positively about ourselves. Compare this to our late inner autumn, when hormones like oestrogen and progesterone are dropping and neurotransmitters like serotonin and dopamine aren't as high as they are earlier in our menstrual cycle, at which time we might not feel as positively disposed to our body.

There has also been a pushback against medical research that primarily uses men as the standard. There are real-world consequences when the impact of cyclical hormonal changes is not factored into research design. Take autoimmune diseases such as rheumatoid arthritis, Alzheimer's and multiple sclerosis. These conditions affect 8 per cent of the global population, 78 per cent of those sufferers are female. In her 2019 book *Doing Harm*, Maya Dusenbery discusses how under-researched and underdiagnosed these conditions are in women, explaining that the research typically focuses on how the symptoms of these conditions appear in men. This often leads to women being taken less seriously when they approach their doctor about their symptoms, and they end up having to wait longer to receive a diagnosis.[4]

When it comes to specific women's health conditions, the conversation is more nuanced. There is still a lack of research into endometriosis, fibroids, adenomyosis and polycystic ovarian syndrome (PCOS). Combine this with the education gap in menstrual and hormone health, and many of us still don't know what to expect when it comes to our period. Think about the culture and religious beliefs we talked about in Chapter 1. If these, along with knowledge gaps and deficits, create confusion about what is normal and what isn't, then my belief is that it's important to put a stake in the ground. This isn't meant to shame anyone for having a period or menstrual cycle that is outside the norm. I'm also not advocating healthism,[5] which places the problem of health and disease in the hands of the individual, rather than acknowledging there are also systemic and political issues – such as the lack of consistent and equitable access to health services, or lack of research into women's health – that contribute to menstrual and hormone health issues.

What I would like to elucidate in this chapter is that there is a healthy continuum when it comes to a normal period and menstrual cycle. This means that you're producing enough oestrogen to build your uterine lining, you're ovulating every cycle, you're making enough progesterone and you're able to continue to live your life even when you have your period.

Contrary to what you may currently believe, if you're outside of this spectrum, there is a way to change things. Later in this book, we explore endometriosis, adenomyosis, fibroids, premenstrual dysphoric disorder (PMDD), PCOS and hypothalamic amenorrhea (HA) – see Chapters 8, 9 and 10.

When I work with my clients in my private practice, I talk to them about what to expect from their period and menstrual cycle, shown in the table below. We then look at where they differ from this norm, what we can do to change this and support their overall hormone and menstrual health.

Menstrual Cycle Length	21–35 days
Period Length	3–7 days
Menstrual Flow	More than 30ml (1.01fl oz), less than 60ml (2.02fl oz) (around 6–7 fully soaked regular tampons or pads, 3–4 full 15ml (0.5fl oz) menstrual cups each period)
Menstrual Colour	Bright red for most of the flow (some dark red toward the end is fine too)
Menstrual Pain	Light cramping, aches
Energy	High during ovulation and low, but not completely exhausted, during menstruation
Ovulation	Midway through cycle, not always on day 14
Cervical Fluid	Changing after menstruation, peak fluid resembles egg white and indicates ovulation
Temperature	Before ovulation: between 36.1°C (96.9°F) and 36.7°C (98°F) Just after ovulation: between 36.4°C (97.5°F) and 37°C (98.6°F)
Mood	More sociable and outgoing during inner spring and summer, less outgoing and more focused during inner autumn and winter

The Role the Menstrual Cycle (and Periods!) Plays in Women's Health

Do we even need to have a period every month? Because so many of us have a hate–hate relationship with our periods for a variety of reasons, we question the need to have a monthly period and menstrual cycle. While we can take the hormonal contraception that stops menstruation, I think it's valuable to consider the role our menstrual cycle plays in our overall health, so we understand that it's about more than just our period!

Without a menstrual cycle, we won't produce enough oestrogen and progesterone, two of the sex hormones that are involved in many of our body's non-reproductive functions and systems. Oestrogen influences our metabolism, vaginal lubrication, bone health, mental health and cognition, libido, cholesterol levels and even how we feel pain! Oestrogen is connected to serotonin levels, so without it, we would see our mood plummet throughout our menstrual cycle.

And then there's progesterone, the incredible anti-inflammatory hormone we produce when we ovulate. It helps calm us and improves our mood by supporting GABA, a brain neurotransmitter that has a sedative-like effect. Progesterone helps us get better sleep, reduces bloating, lowers blood pressure, improves the function of our thyroid and has a protective effect on our breast tissue.

I know that some of you reading this book may be on hormonal contraception, for a variety of reasons. What you might not know is that the synthetic hormones in the Pill, the Mirena coil, the Nuva Ring and other forms of hormonal contraception are not the same as the ones we make ourselves. I want to be clear that there is no judgement from me about your choice to use hormonal contraception. It's your choice. Do not let anyone shame you for it. In my private clinic, I always ask my clients to make sure they're making an *informed* choice, where they understand both the benefits and side effects of what they're taking. For example, for those with endometriosis, short-term hormonal contraception prescribed by their doctor can be helpful, as it shuts off oestrogen and progesterone production. This then helps us deal with the inflammation and gut issues at the heart of many endo symptoms. In the long term, there are downsides to hormonal contraception that aren't often discussed, including loss of libido, mood changes (including depression), struggling to get your period back (called post-Pill amenorrhea) and potential fertility issues. Unfortunately, there are currently very few studies looking at the long-term effect of hormonal contraception.

If you are considering coming off hormonal contraception, please speak to your doctor. Some of my clients become

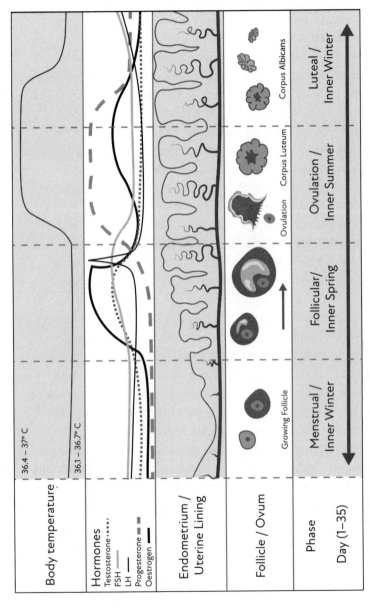

What's Happening During the Menstrual Cycle

disillusioned by the return of their original symptoms after coming off hormonal contraception, something I call the boomerang effect. This is a sign that your body needs support to address the root cause of your original symptoms, as well as support to address the nutrient deficiencies created by using hormonal contraception. If this is you, the book *Beyond The Pill* (2019) by Dr Jolene Brighten is a great resource.

Are You More Stressed Than You Realize?

Have you ever been told to lower your stress levels and thought, "Okay, I know that, but how?" It's become a truism that we should all reduce stress. Many of us are more stressed than we realize, and this ongoing stress has a negative effect on menstrual health.

Let me back up a bit. The stressors, or causes of stress, we experience can be physical (excessive exercise, not eating enough, not getting or absorbing enough nutrients from the food you eat), emotional / mental (issues with work, family, friends) or even external (pollution, climate change, racism). Our nervous system helps us respond to and manage the impact of the different stressors we experience. Our nervous system is split into two parts: the central and peripheral nervous systems. The central nervous system includes all the nerves in the brain and spine, while the nerves in the rest of the body, including the skeletal system, are part of the peripheral nervous system. There are nerves that we have voluntary control over, such as those that allow us to blink our eyes or move our fingers to turn the pages of this book. This is the somatic nervous system.[6] Then there are the parts of the nervous system we don't have control over, and these make up the autonomic nervous system (ANS). The ANS regulates how fast our heart beats, how quickly we digest food, even sexual arousal. When we talk about the effects of stress, we're most interested in the autonomic nervous system, which we can then split into the sympathetic (SNS) and parasympathetic nervous systems (PNS). The table below breaks out what happens when each part of the ANS is activated.

Sympathetic Nervous System (SNS)	Parasympathetic Nervous System (PNS)
Fight, flight, freeze, fawn	Rest, digest, tend, befriend
The body responds to a perceived threat	The body feels safe
Slowed digestion	Improved digestion
Increased heartbeat	Heartbeat regulates and slows
Pupils dilate for extreme focus	Pupils constrict
Increased adrenaline and cortisol release	Adrenaline and cortisol levels normalize
Increased insulin release from the pancreas	Insulin levels normalize

In an ideal world, we would all have good autonomic tone, meaning we can easily shift between the sympathetic and parasympathetic nervous systems, using our breath and other tools to tell our bodies that we're safe and there is no threat. This autonomic tone would also help us identify when we're experiencing good stress (eustress) and bad stress (distress). Good stress is the anticipation of going on holiday and feeling excited about what you need to do to prepare for it. Bad stress is making a pre-holiday to-do list and feeling panicked and overwhelmed by everything on it. I explore this in more detail in Chapter 6.

Bringing us back to the effects of stress on our menstrual health, we need to look at what's happening in our brains. Our stress response system is governed by the HPA axis, which stands for hypothalamus (the hormone control centre in our brains), pituitary gland (a gland in our brain that releases hormones) and adrenals (tiny hormone glands that sit on top of our kidneys). When we are overly distressed, it's the connection between these three organs that leads to chronic cortisol production. Remember, cortisol is our primary stress hormone and this is released when our bodies are in an extended time of stress. When we produce too much cortisol, it inhibits gonadotropin-releasing hormone (GnRH), the hormone that tells our pituitary gland to release follicle stimulating hormone (FSH) and luteinizing hormone (LH). This will have a negative effect on our menstrual health in several ways, including changes in length of the menstrual cycle and period. At its worst, severe stress can stop periods altogether, which I explore in more detail in Chapter 10.

What We Eat Helps Support Menstrual Health

As you'll discover, the food we eat every day can be incredibly beneficial for our menstrual and hormone health. You'll learn about foods that help during each of the four phases of the menstrual cycle. But before we get into this, we need to cover the basics.

This is always one of the first things I examine with my clients. I evaluate how often they're eating and gently encourage them to move away from skipping meals, overly restrictive intermittent-fasting regimes and excessive snacking. We look at each of the three meals most of us eat each day and then build from there. I always start from a place of addition, rather than subtraction, thinking of what they can add to each meal to make it even more beneficial for their menstrual and hormone health. They discover that simple tweaks can make a big difference, especially over the long term.

In a world that so often asks that we restrict and make ourselves smaller, I love showing my clients what they can add, rather than subtract. Likewise, you won't find a discussion of being gluten-, sugar- or dairy-free in this book. Of course, for some people, removing these foods can be beneficial, but if these foods are causing an issue, that's a sign of a deeper issue that won't be solved by simply cutting them out forever.

I always recommend working with a qualified nutritionist who can help you run functional testing such as stool or urine tests to get to the bottom of your health concerns.

Equally, you won't find an emphasis on a particular eating regime here. I'll say to you what I say to my clients: you have to eat in a way that makes you feel good, gives you lots of energy, supports your mood and contributes to good menstrual and hormone health. For some of us, this means eating red meat, and for others, this means eating using a vegetarian or vegan template. Some of my clients have found that they have more energy and lighter periods after adding a little more high-quality red meat, while some clients have found that adding more plant-based protein and simply eating more vegetables has been beneficial for them. If you notice that you don't feel great after eating a particular type of food, that's a sign that you need to investigate further.

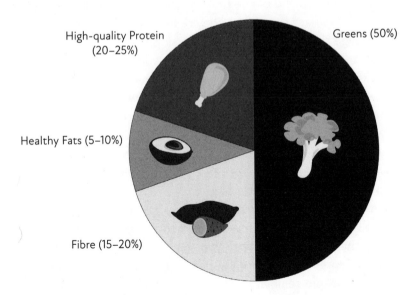

High-quality Protein (20–25%)

Greens (50%)

Healthy Fats (5–10%)

Fibre (15–20%)

How to Build a Balanced Plate

So where should you start? Let's begin with the four basics I like to build each meal around: high-quality protein, healthy fats, greens and fibre. We'll get into the why for each element shortly, but at the heart of this combination is support for balanced blood sugar levels, the ingredients for making the hormones you need and getting the nutrients you need to support a healthy menstrual cycle.

High-quality Protein

Free-range, organic red meat, poultry, eggs and dairy, wild fish and seafood, beans, lentils, chickpeas/garbanzo beans, fermented tofu, tempeh and miso.

Every time I go to the grocery store, it seems like there's another product screaming about all the protein it contains and how it will help build muscle. Yes, protein does help build muscle (and this becomes a bigger consideration after 30, when we start to lose 3 to 8 per cent of muscle mass each year),[7] but there are other benefits, especially for our menstrual cycle, that I would rather focus on.

We need to make sure we're eating enough protein to support blood sugar balance. Supporting your blood sugar means eating enough at each meal to feel satiated, so you have enough energy to get you to your next meal and your mood remains stable. Like fat, we do most of our protein digestion in our stomach, so it's slower to break down compared to a piece of fruit or bread, which starts breaking down in our mouths as we're chewing it. The longer food takes to digest, the more stable our blood sugar levels.

The amino acids – such as tryptophan,[8] tyrosine and phenylalanine[9] – that group together to form protein also form the building blocks of the feel-good neurotransmitters like serotonin and dopamine and peptide hormones like FSH, thyroxine (T4), adrenaline, oxytocin, melatonin and insulin. Vital organs like the liver and thyroid need protein to function well. Our liver is where we break down protein into amino acids and convert amino acids into glucose, fat and proteins. We need protein, specifically the amino acid tyrosine from our food, to help the inactive thyroid hormone T4 convert to the active thyroid hormone T3 in the liver, gut and muscles, as well as to make the protein thyroglobulin, which helps us make T4 and T3.[10] We'll talk about the importance of the thyroid and our menstrual cycle later in this chapter.

We also need more protein at different points in our menstrual cycle. A 2016 American study found that the women participating increased their protein intake, specifically with animal protein, in the luteal phase, due to increased appetite levels from rising progesterone.[11] We'll dive deeper into this in Chapter 7, where we discuss the luteal phase. Throughout your menstrual cycle, try to make sure that 20 to 25 per cent of each meal is composed of protein.

Healthy Fats
Oily fish (I love the acronym SMASHHT to remember these: sardines, mackerel, anchovies, salmon, haddock, herring, trout), nuts, seeds, nut butters, butter, ghee, olive oil, avocados, avocado oils, full-fat coconut milk and cream.

Growing up in the 1990s and early 2000s, I remember flipping through magazines where dietary fat was portrayed as the enemy. Butter was bad and margarine was in! When I first started my clinical nutrition practice, I spent a lot of time unpicking the bias against fat and re-educating my clients about the importance of dietary fat. When I discuss eating fat, I find that there is often a need to discuss fears around gaining weight and fatphobia. *Fearing the Black Body: The Racial Origins of Fat Phobia* by Sabrina Strings is a great book if you want to delve more into this topic.

Think about the way you eat. Do you ever find yourself veering toward low-fat options in the grocery store? I would love for you to read this section and start to unlearn some of these behaviours. Fat is a rich source of energy and is what makes our food taste so good. Look at yogurt as an example. Low-fat versions typically add sugar to increase the flavour profile, whereas full-fat yogurt is delicious on its own.

Like protein, fat triggers satiety hormones, which help you feel full.[12] Although we have enzymes in our saliva that break down some fat, much like that of protein, digestion of fat really kicks off in the stomach, which means that including this in your meals is another way to help balance your blood sugar levels and keep your mood stable. Additionally, without enough fat in our meals, we would have trouble absorbing and using the important fat-soluble vitamins A, D, E and K. The fat we get in our food also supports the health of our brain, nervous system, skin, eyes, hair and even our mental health.

When it comes to our hormones, we need to eat fat to make some of the ones that guide our menstrual cycle: pregnanolone, cortisol, oestrogen, progesterone, testosterone and DHEA. These are examples of steroid hormones, hormones created from cholesterol,[13] some of which comes from dietary sources.[14]

There's a lot of controversy around dietary fat and I'll do my best in this section to steer you in the right direction. When in doubt, focus on whole-food sources of fat such as oily fish, butter, coconut, avocados, nuts and seeds.

Not all dietary fat is created equal and it's easy to fall into a trap of calling all saturated fats unhealthy and all unsaturated fats healthy. There's nuance here, and without acknowledging this, we risk losing out on the benefits of many amazing foods! The chart on the next two pages breaks down the complicated world of dietary fat.

Fats that have seemingly been written off, such as those in butter, coconut and red meat (which is a mix of protein and fat), have benefits beyond their fat content. This is why it's important to move away from reductionist thinking that demonizes foods. If you say all red meat is bad because of

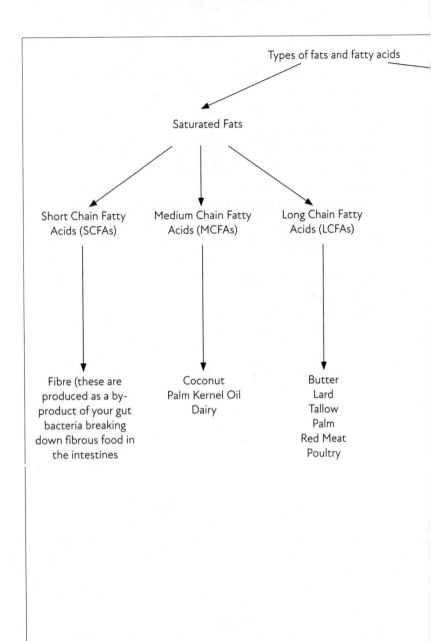

The World of Dietary Fat

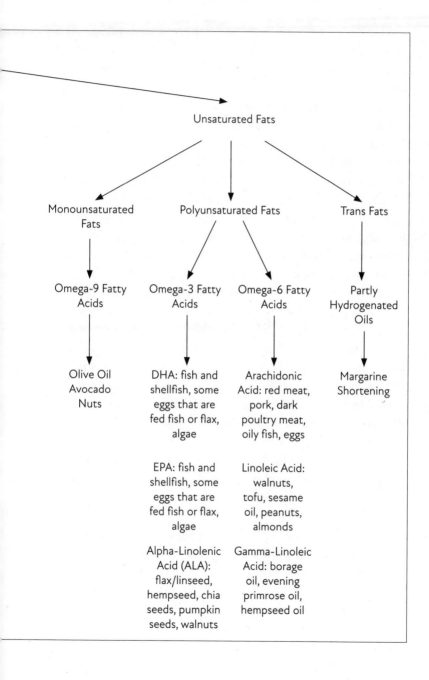

the fat it contains, you miss out on the iron, zinc, vitamin A, B vitamins and more. My only caveat here is artificial trans-fatty acids. I highly recommend avoiding foods such as margarine and shortening because they can increase the risk of heart disease and raise inflammatory markers in the body.[15]

Some fats, which we call essential fatty acids (EFAs), can only be obtained through food. These EFAs are omega-3 and omega-6 fatty acids. Omega-3 fatty acids such as eicosapentaenoic acid (EPA) and docosahexaenoic acid (DHA) are primarily found in oily fish and algae. These fatty acids are powerful anti-inflammatories, incredibly important for our brains to work well and the way our nervous system functions. They also make up the fatty layer on the outside of our cells, including the ovum, the mature egg that's released at ovulation (which is the biggest cell in the body!).

We don't just need to eat fish to get omega-3 fatty acids. They're also in foods such as flax, hemp, chia and pumpkin seeds. Do note that they contain a form of omega-3 called alpha-linolenic acid (ALA), which doesn't convert as well to DHA and EPA, so I typically advise my clients to use a good fish oil or algae (for the vegans) supplement to make sure they're getting enough omega-3 fatty acids.

Just like with protein, we need more fat at various points in our menstrual cycle. During the early luteal phase, when our progesterone levels are still high, our body's ability to break down fat and protein increases,[16] which can then increase our appetite. Fats contain a lot of energy, so a little goes a long way. Throughout your menstrual cycle, try to make sure around 5 to 10 per cent of each meal is composed of healthy fats.

WHAT COOKING OIL SHOULD I USE?

Oddly enough, this is a question I get asked all the time. I once gave an hour-long menstrual health workshop where we inadvertently spent 30 minutes talking about cooking oils and the bewilderment around them! There is a lot of confusion about which fats we should use to cook our foods. I hope this will help break it down for you. All fats have something called a smoke point, which is the highest temperature it can be heated to before it starts to oxidize and burn. I always recommend using oils with a high smoke point for cooking, especially when you're doing high-temperature tasks like roasting, searing, browning, frying and sautéing. I don't recommend cooking with the following oils: vegetable, corn, rapeseed/canola and sunflower. These are all high in omega-6, which can be inflammatory when there is no omega-3 to balance it out. These oils are typically sold in clear plastic or glass bottles, indicating that they have already started to oxidize by the time you take them home and start cooking. These oils are also highly processed – extracted using chemical solvents, bleached and then deodorized.

Remember, all oils break down eventually, so use what you have within 60 to 90 days. Keep all your cooking fats in the cupboard, as exposure to light will oxidize them, reduce their benefits and increase their inflammatory potential. Try to buy oils in a dark bottle because this helps protect them from oxidization.

Cooking Fat Smoke Points

Cooking Fat	Smoke Point
Avocado oil	266°C (511°F)
Ghee	252°C (486°F)
Coconut oil	205°C (401°F)
Macadamia nut oil	199°C (390°F)
Duck fat	190°C (374°F)
Extra virgin olive oil	190°C (374°F)
Butter	145°C (293°F)

Greens

Kale, broccoli, Brussels sprouts, pak choi/bok choy, cauliflower, broccoli rabe, swede/rutabaga leaves, spring/collard greens, kohlrabi, okra, beetroot/beet greens, rocket/arugula, watercress, winter greens, microgreens, spinach, cos/romaine lettuce, chard, chicory/endive, radicchio, cabbage.

I'll admit it: I love kale. I'm a total nutrition cliché and I must give a shout-out to kale's publicist. They did a fantastic job! Kale aside, I love it when my clients add more green vegetables into their meals. These are full of fibre, which we'll talk more about in the next section, and they have an array of amazing benefits for our liver, gut and hormones.

When it comes to supporting hormones, it's so valuable to do what you can to support your liver and gut. Both organs help our bodies detoxify, or break down, hormones like oestrogen once we've used them. Yes, our body can detoxify itself without the need for special teas and shakes, but there are certain nutrients and nutritional compounds that help this process along.

Many of the greens above are in a family of vegetables called crucifers. These vegetables contain plant compounds that support the liver during the three-phase process it goes through to break down hormones like oestrogen before they get eliminated through bowel movements.[17] For more detail about this process, flip to Chapter 8.

Unless you've had it removed, I bet you've never really thought about your gallbladder. Greens are a fantastic way to support the gallbladder, the organ beneath our liver that produces bile. Once it goes from the gallbladder to the liver, bile is used to break down and digest dietary fat. The bitter taste in green vegetables like crucifers comes from a family of plant compounds called glucosinolates.[18] These stimulate the gallbladder to produce bile, which also helps our body better utilize the fat-soluble vitamins, A, D, E and K.

These vegetables are also a fantastic source of B vitamins, which are important for menstrual and hormone health. When you put your plate together, aim for half of it to be made up of these green vegetables. If that's too much, could you add a new-to-you green vegetable to your dinners this week? And another next week? Keep building until it becomes second nature for you to have loads of greens on your plate.

Fibre

Beans, lentils, chickpeas/garbanzo beans, nuts, seeds, quinoa, fruits and vegetables with the skin still on them, whole grains, brown rice, brown pasta, sweet potatoes, carrots, broccoli, cauliflower, squash, pumpkin, swede/rutabaga.

When I was growing up, fibre equalled prunes / dried plums, Bran Flakes and Metamucil (which is just psyllium husk capsules!). In Canada, television commercials told us we needed to include fibre to keep us regular, but failed to mention the most easily accessed source of fibre: fruits and vegetables.

Along with protein and fat, fibre supports blood sugar balance,[19] taking us off the rollercoaster that can lead to us craving sweets or feeling hangry and tired. Our gut bacteria, the little critters that live in our small and large intestine, feed off the fibre in our food. What's cool about this process is that the by-product of fibrous fermentation produces short-chain fatty acids (SCFAs). We have three major SCFAs, called butyrate, acetate and propionate, all of which play a role in the interaction between our gut and brain. They have a beneficial effect on the health of the gut itself, help to reduce inflammation and positively impact brain function and mood.[20]

Fibre supports our menstrual and hormone health by helping us have regular bowel movements. When I was studying, one of my lecturers commented that we should be aiming for three bowel movements a day, and I've never forgotten that. Every bowel movement we have helps us eliminate waste, including the hormones our liver and gut have broken down through the process of detoxification. When we're constipated, these hormones have nowhere to go and can recirculate back into the body. This is bad news if you have any issues with your menstrual health – such as premenstrual symptoms or painful or heavy periods – as constipation can exacerbate these issues.

When it comes to the composition of your plate, making it about 15 to 20 per cent fibre is helpful for all of the benefits we've just discussed. This will help you get to the NHS's recommendation of 30g of fibre each day.[21]

What About Carbohydrates?

You'll notice that I haven't mentioned carbohydrates. You do need to eat carbohydrates for healthy periods; but I find there is a stigma around carbs and I spend a lot of time unpicking this with my clients. By refocusing on greens and fibre, we reframe the understanding of carbohydrates to focus on their benefits.

When it comes down to it, carbohydrates are just chains of sugar of varying levels of complexity: monosaccharides, disaccharides and polysaccharides. You might know them as simple or complex carbohydrates. Would it surprise you to know that fruits and vegetables are carbohydrates? There are so many benefits to these foods – their fibre, vitamins and minerals – that when we focus on them as just chains of sugar, we lose out on all of their other advantages. For example, we need to eat carbohydrates to support thyroid hormone conversion in the gut and liver.

A word on fruit in particular: you may hear some in the health and wellbeing space saying that natural fructose (a type of sugar) is bad for us and that we should avoid high-sugar fruit. I don't agree with this at all. Bananas are an example of a high-sugar fruit. They are also packed with potassium, which helps reduce premenstrual bloating, and fibre, which helps us have daily bowel movements. What about pineapples? They are much maligned as too high in sugar; but they are another high-fibre fruit that also contains bromelain, an enzyme with anti-inflammatory effects that helps us digest protein.[22] These examples illustrate yet another reason why it's crucial to avoid a reductionist view of the foods you eat.

Don't Forget About Water

How much water have you drunk today? It's such a basic health tip, but sometimes we all need a reminder of the importance of the basics, right? There's a lot of debate in the health world about the right amount of water to drink each day. Some say 2l (4 pints), some say 1.5l (3 pints). Here's what I say to my clients: if you're eating a wide variety of fruits and vegetables each day, you'll be absorbing water from them. Then all you need to do is top up according to your thirst levels. You don't need to down water all day, especially right before and during meals, because this will dilute your digestive juices, affecting your stomach's ability to effectively break down the food you eat. Overhydration is just as bad as underhydration, putting too much pressure on your kidneys and reducing sodium and potassium levels.

Throughout this book, I talk about the role of the gut and liver in supporting menstrual and hormone health. The kidneys are another key player. Drinking enough water helps us have healthy kidneys. We want this because the kidneys activate vitamin D, a hormone that helps reduce period pain, supports ovulation and improves bone health. Our kidneys are also where we make prostaglandins, the hormone-like compounds that are responsible for many functions, including the contractions that help us shed the lining of our uterus when we have our periods. Through our urine, we also excrete some of the oestrogens that have been used and broken down by our body.[23]

So how much water should you drink? You want to make sure that your urine isn't dark yellow or completely colourless. Aim for a very light yellow. And if you take a multivitamin (ideally in the morning, so the B vitamins which help us produce energy don't affect your sleep), the riboflavin, or B2, might make your urine a bright yellow. This is normal and nothing to worry about.

A Word on the Thyroid

Would it surprise you to learn that the health of our thyroid (the butterfly-shaped gland at the base of the front of our throat) has a direct impact on our menstrual cycle, ovulation and sex hormones like oestrogen and progesterone?

The thyroid influences so many systems in our body. It regulates the body's metabolic rate, which means it controls how hot or cold we are, the speed we digest our food, even how quickly our heart beats!

We produce two hormones: thyrotropin-releasing hormone (TRH) and thyroid-stimulating hormone (TSH) from our brain, which then encourage our thyroid to release T4 (the inactive thyroid hormone) and T3 (the active thyroid hormone). The body brings in the kidneys, liver and the gut to help convert T4 to T3, which is another example of how nothing in the body works in isolation. A healthy gut (our small and large intestine) and liver are important for how much oestrogen and progesterone we have available for our body to use, as well as for the health of our thyroid.

You might be thinking: "I thought this was a book about periods! Why are you talking about the thyroid?" Bear with me. There is a fantastic interplay between our thyroid and its hormones and our ovaries, uterus and sex hormones. We have thyroid hormone (T4 and T3) receptors on our ovaries and uterus, and these affect the development and metabolism of these important organs.[24] We also have oestrogen receptors (remember the lock-and-key mechanism for hormones and neurotransmitters we talked about in the last chapter?) on our thyroid.[25] This means that the amount of oestrogen in our body influences the health of our thyroid. Like Goldilocks, we want to have just the right amount of oestrogen relative to where we are in our menstrual cycle, because it helps our body make thyroglobulin, a protein stored in the thyroid that gets broken down whenever our body needs T4 and T3.

When we have too much oestrogen in relation to progesterone, the liver produces more thyroglobulin, which binds to our thyroid hormones and decreases the amount available for the body to use. This isn't good news because we need enough thyroid hormone for our thyroid to work properly.

When we don't have enough oestrogen, this has a negative effect on the thyroid itself, because oestrogen stimulates thyroid growth and, as we've seen above, is involved in supporting our body's need for T4 and T3.

We also need to consider the thyroid's effect on progesterone. Not enough thyroid hormone affects our ability to ovulate and make progesterone.[26] This can lead to a variety of symptoms, including heavier periods, premenstrual spotting, missing periods, lighter periods and premenstrual mood changes. We want to have enough progesterone because this helps positively increase the amount of thyroid hormone in the blood and increases its ability to get into our body's cells for them to use. And remember, we make progesterone when we ovulate. For more on ovulation, flip to Chapter 6.

The interplay I've just described is why I always investigate the thyroid when my clients come to me with any menstrual health issue. It's easy to simply say that someone has a heavy period, but we always want to try to understand the cause. This means considering whether thyroid issues are negatively impacting menstrual health.

The thyroid is a delicate gland, and we want to make sure it's just right (remember Goldilocks!). When the thyroid is underactive or not making enough thyroid hormone, this is called hypothyroidism, of which there is a spectrum, ranging from subclinical (the thyroid is ever so slightly underactive) to primary (a fully underactive thyroid). There is also an autoimmune component to this, called Hashimoto's thyroiditis, where thyroid antibodies (special proteins that attach to foreign invaders in the body) attack the thyroid gland.

On the flip side, the thyroid can be overactive, producing high levels of T4 and T3 and low levels of TSH. As with hypothyroidism, there is a spectrum from subclinical to primary hyperthyroidism. Graves' disease is the autoimmune version of hyperthyroidism. A nodule on the thyroid, which produces excess thyroid hormone, can also cause hyperthyroidism.

Signs and Symptoms of Hypothyroidism and Hyperthyroidism

Hypothyroidism[27]	Hyperthyroidism[28]
General Signs and Symptoms	
Cold hands and feet	Rapid pulse, breathlessness (please phone 999 in the UK and 911 in the US if you feel either of these symptoms!)
Struggling to get warm, even in the summer	Excessive sweating, warm and moist skin
Constipation	Frequent bowel movements
Unexplained weight gain / struggling to lose weight	Unexplained weight loss, increased appetite
Hair loss / dry, thinning hair	Fine, brittle hair and nails
Dry skin	Bulging eyes
Memory and concentration issues	Inability to concentrate
Excessive fatigue	Restlessness, difficulty sleeping
Puffy face	Swelling at the base of the neck, due to a goitre (an enlarged thyroid gland)
Low moods and depression	Twitching / trembling
Difficulty conceiving	Difficulty conceiving
Weakness and aches in muscles and joints	Muscle weakness
Menstrual Signs and Symptoms	
Heavy periods	Missing periods
Irregular periods	Irregular periods
Premenstrual spotting	Light periods
Ovarian cysts	Very short luteal phase
Light periods	
Anovulation (menstrual cycles with no ovulation)	

How to Get Your Thyroid Checked

If you've read this section and you have at least three to four of the symptoms of either hypo or hyperthyroidism, I strongly encourage you to get your thyroid tested. In my clinical experience, I've seen that some doctors will only check TSH and T4. You must push them to at least test T3 as well, so you have a more complete picture of your thyroid health. If this isn't possible, there are a wide range of private testing options available.

Here are the ranges I use in my clinic for thyroid results. You may notice that these ranges are different to what you may see in your NHS blood test report. In my clinical experience, I find these functional ranges are where my clients feel their best. They'll help us thrive, not just stay alive.

My top tip is to get your thyroid tested in the morning if possible, as we produce most of our thyroid hormones in the early hours.[29]

	Why Test This?	Optimal Reference Range
TSH	To assess your pituitary gland's ability to make enough thyroid hormone	1–2mIU/l
Free T4	To assess levels of thyroid hormone circulating in the body	15–23pmol/l
Free T3	To assess levels of active thyroid hormone circulating in the body and if you're converting T4 correctly	3.4–6.0pmol/l
Reverse T3	To assess how much free T3 can bind to thyroid receptors	11–18ng/dl
Thyroid peroxidase (TPO)	To assess if the autoimmune version of hypothyroidism or hyperthyroidism is present	<35kIU/l
Thyroglobulin antibodies (TgAB)	To assess if the autoimmune version of hypothyroidism or hyperthyroidism is present	<30kIU/l

	Why Test This?	Optimal Reference Range
Thyroid-stimulating immunoglobulin (TSI)	To assess if the autoimmune version of hyperthyroidism is present	<0.55IU/l
TSH receptor antibodies (TRAb)	To assess if the autoimmune version of hyperthyroidism is present	16–100 per cent inhibition of TSH binding

Arika's Story

Arika's first period arrived with a bang, not a whimper. She vividly remembers the day it started. She woke up like she did every day, looking forward to seeing her friends at school and maybe chatting with her crush, Tom. In maths, her stomach started feeling strange, a stabbing pain that seemed to increase in intensity over the course of the school day. She tried to get through the day as best as she could, but after lunch, she decided to go to the nurse's office. Before she got there, Arika noticed her underwear felt wet and was mortified to think she might have peed her pants. She ran to the bathroom and found a strange red patch in her underwear. The nurse kindly told Arika her period had arrived.

For years, Arika could predict her cycle like clockwork. She would have two great weeks and then two terrible weeks. She was a mess the week before her period: crying at the drop of a hat, mainlining chocolate and using heavy-duty foundation to cover up the hormonal acne on her chin and jaw. And then there was the week of her period. Day 1 and 2 were always a write-off and she would do as little as possible, using painkillers to deal with her little stabby friend, as she called her period pain.

Like many of my clients, Arika had had enough by the time we started working together. Arika's menstrual health didn't change overnight. Think of it like building a house. We wanted to make sure the foundations were solid: getting enough sleep, eating meals that included a diverse range of greens, fibre, high-quality protein and healthy fats, regular exercise and movement, nervous system support and strong connections with the community around her. And supplements were the cherry on top of the cake that helped Arika change her menstrual and hormone health a little faster.

Now, Arika's period and menstrual health are what I would describe as normal: her cycle is regular, she feels in control of her emotions and cravings in the week before her period and her period is less heavy, with the odd cramps and twinge. And importantly, Arika knows that her period is not perfect (does anyone have a *perfect* period?!), but she knows what she can do to continue to have a normal period.

In the next four chapters, I'll navigate you through what's happening during each phase of the menstrual cycle, so that by the time you read to the end of this section, you'll understand the biological, physical, hormonal and mental / cognitive changes that take place. As ever, I encourage you to use this information to guide you, rather than to let yourself feel restricted by it. We're never aiming for perfection. Go through the book and pick a few things that resonate for you, add them into your daily routine in a way that feels sustainable. For more about building sustainable habits, check out the books in the Resources (see pages 297–302).

You'll learn how to support your cyclical nature and, perhaps, even use it to your advantage!

PART 2

Phases of the Menstrual Cycle

CHAPTER 4

The Menstrual Phase / Inner Winter

Periods. The time of the month. Aunt Flo. The blob. Surfing the crimson wave. The Reds. Whatever you call your period, for most of us, this is the time in our menstrual cycles that looms large. In the next four chapters, I'll be taking you through each of the four phases of the menstrual cycle, beginning with where we start each cycle: menstruation, aka your period / menses / menstrual phase.

Sarah's Story

Sarah said her periods were taking over her life. She had gone from periods that were five days long, painless, fairly light and came every 30 days like clockwork to what she described as endless periods that could last up to 14 days and were extremely heavy and painful.

Sarah said that, for her, the most startling change was going from never really thinking about her period to structuring her entire life around it. Her energy levels were through the floor, she was irritable and always tired. When she first came to see me in clinic, she described herself as being at the end of her tether. She felt like I was her very last resort. When I heard

PHASES OF THE MENSTRUAL CYCLE

that, I knew I had to find a way to help her make changes that would have a quick effect on her energy and mood, while also helping Sarah create sustainable lifestyle and nutrition habits.

Sarah had been to see her doctor but felt as though all they wanted to do was put her on the Pill and give her some iron tablets. She didn't want to go on the Pill and was keen to find a way to get to the root cause of what was going on with her heavy periods and get her life back.

I'm sure you can relate to parts of Sarah's story.

We started by looking at what Sarah was eating, discussing the importance of iron and how those of us with heavy bleeds can lose on average 1.4mg of iron through our menstrual fluid each day during our periods.[1] For context, we need to obtain about 14.8mg through our food each day. Sarah had had heavy periods for at least five years. In this time, she had also found herself eating less and less red meat, for a variety of reasons, and she was never able to build up her iron levels enough to replace what was lost during her period. This contributed to her ongoing feeling of endless fatigue.

After her blood tests came back, with her doctor confirming severe iron deficiency anaemia, I recommended a short-term, high-quality iron bisglycinate supplement to quickly increase her levels, with added vitamin C to boost absorption. We had a chat about her drift toward vegetarianism and she agreed that she felt comfortable with adding in free-range, organic red meat from her local farm at least three times a week. (P.S. Don't worry if you're reading this and would never consider eating meat. I've got you covered in the iron section on page 84). We also added in vegetarian sources of iron and vitamin C, as well as foods containing copper and vitamin A to help her body better use the iron she was getting from food and supplements.

We then moved on to address what in her diet and lifestyle could be causing the chronic inflammation that was leading to her painful periods. Chronic inflammation occurs when the body's defence mechanism, the immune system, acts as though there is a continued threat it needs to respond to.[2] As we'll find out later in this chapter, a number of things result in chronic inflammation. In Sarah's case, we identified high sugar intake, alcohol binges and high work stress as the main drivers of the chronic inflammation she was experiencing. To address this, we started by making her meals more nourishing with more fibre, more high-quality protein and healthy fats to balance her blood sugar levels and reduce her sweet cravings.

Sarah had got into the habit of having a couple of large glasses of wine every night with dinner. We talked about a more mindful approach to drinking alcohol, including avoiding binge drinking, which isn't just having lots of shots. Binge drinking is also drinking several large glasses of wine, which is nearly a whole bottle! Have a look at how regularly you're drinking and how much you drink when you do. Do you drink every day? Alcohol has a hugely negative impact on our menstrual and hormone health due to its effect on our liver, which has to turn it to acetaldehyde, a toxic substance, in order for it to be cleared from the body.[3] This means that the liver wants to get rid of it as soon as possible, so it prioritizes this over its other functions, including breaking down the hormones our body has used. When my clients reduce their alcohol intake, it usually has a positive effect on their menstrual and hormone health. My view is that we need to have an honest conversation about drinking.

Binge drinking in its many forms (wine o'clock, happy hour, bottomless brunch) has been normalized, without a corresponding conversation about the effect it has on our health, periods and hormones. If you'd like to read more about this, try the books listed on page 328.

To combat some of the effects stress might be having on her system, I asked her to practise box breathing at least five to six times a day to help manage her nervous system and get her out of fight or flight mode, which was increasing her cortisol levels (see page 99). Managing our nervous system is an essential part of improving our menstrual health. It's not just as simple as reducing stress. We need to manage a part of our nervous system called the autonomic nervous system. This is split into two parts: sympathetic (fight or flight) and parasympathetic (rest, digest, tend and befriend). When we're stuck in fight or flight through chronic stress, cortisol, our primary stress hormone, increases. This negatively affects our blood sugar balance because cortisol is a catabolic hormone, releasing sugar in the blood for energy. This can lead to blood sugar crashes and compounds existing fatigue.

When she came to see me a month later, Sarah reported that her last period was a little lighter and her pain levels dropped from a self-evaluated score of 8 out of 10 to a 5 out of 10. Over the next three months, we continued to layer on different foods and lifestyle changes that would support her hormonal and menstrual health. After another three months, we retested her iron levels and they were back into the normal range, her self-reported pain levels were now between 3–5 out of 10 and she was bleeding much less during her period. Sarah said that she was feeling less fatigued and irritable, and felt that she could maintain these changes for the long term.

Delving into Our Menstrual Phase / Inner Winter

Let's delve deeper into exactly what happens during the menstrual phase of our cycle, which starts on day 1 of our periods. What we like to think of as a normal period can last from 3 to 7 days. As I talked about in Chapter 2, our periods are what we tend to focus on when we think about our menstrual cycles, predominantly due to the negative experiences many of us have had with them, including painful periods and mood changes, which I explore in Chapters 8 and 9 of this book.

But it's no wonder we tend to focus so much on our periods: they form a huge part of our life experience. We have them for between 35 and 41 years of our lives, depending on how old we are when our periods start and how old we are when we have our last period (we're considered to be in menopause when we haven't had a period for 12 months). That's an average of 450 periods during our menstruating years. Across the world, the average girl starts menstruating at around 12 or 13 years old, although research shows that the age of menarche (the first menstruation) is happening earlier and earlier, with some girls starting at eight or nine years old, depending on their race and ethnicity.[4] According to the NHS, the average age for girls in the UK to start puberty is 11 years old.[5]

Given how often we get them and how long they last, it makes sense that our periods have a big impact on our lives. But it doesn't have to be negative. As I go through each phase of the menstrual cycle in this book and help you navigate some of the issues you may be experiencing, I hope that you'll gradually shift the way you see your period – you might even see it as something positive. If positivity is a bridge too far (I get it!), then even just feeling neutral about the whole thing is a great place to be.

Before you picked up this book, did you think of your menstrual bleed and your menstrual cycle as the same thing? I know I used to. I didn't learn much about periods in school, I only cobbled things together from reading about it on the internet, in magazines and speaking to friends, who, to be honest, didn't really have a clue themselves.

As we've seen, the American College of Obstetricians and Gynecologists recommends thinking of our menstrual cycle as one of our vital signs,[6] deeming it just as important as blood pressure, pulse / heart rate, breath or respiration rate and body temperature for evaluating overall health status. Looking at our menstrual cycles includes our period, as well as ovulation. If we're not having a period and ovulating each cycle, it can have a detrimental effect on our health, physically and emotionally. I'll talk more about this in Chapter 6.

Many women I've spoken to consider their period to be their menstrual cycle and have no awareness of, or connection to, the rest of their menstrual cycle. I've lost count of the number of women I speak to who call their periods their cycles and then look at me quizzically when I talk about what might be happening for them during the rest of the menstrual cycle. I want all of us to understand that *menstruation is wholly connected to and influenced by the rest of the menstrual cycle* and vice versa, and the whole thing exists in a wonderful healthy circle, if everything is going well. This means that everything we do, including what we eat and drink, our stress levels, our quality of sleep and our connections with our community during the other three phases of our menstrual cycle can have a positive or negative effect on our experience of menstruation itself.

For example, did you do a lot of binge drinking / recreational drugs one month? You may feel and see the negative effects of that on your next one to three periods. Or are you starting to add in more vegetables like broccoli, Brussels sprouts and kale into your meals? You might see the positive effects of this in gentler, less painful periods over your next two to three periods.

As a vital sign, our menstrual cycle, including the menstrual phase (our period), is sensitive to *everything* that's happening in our lives: what we eat, how we move, how stressed we are, our environment, what we put on and in our bodies – *even the way we speak to ourselves* has an effect.

Let's put this into context. Although it takes about a year for a follicle (which is an oocyte, or immature egg cell surrounded by a layer of granulosa cells)[7] to grow into an ovum, or a mature egg, through a process called folliculogenesis,[8] there are stages to this process. Our lifestyle and nutrition affect this whole process. However, when it comes to menstrual health, we typically focus on the 70 days the mature, or antral, ovarian follicle takes to develop enough to be ready for ovulation.[9] What we do during this time can impact the growth of that mature egg, as well the amount of progesterone that's released from the corpus luteum, the structure that is left over after the egg moves out of the ovary into the fallopian tube during ovulation. The more progesterone we produce, the calmer we'll feel during the lead-up to our periods. We'll get into this in detail in Chapter 6.

We're physiologically impacted by the amount of stress we're under, the type of food we eat and the amount of alcohol and drugs we take. These contribute to inflammation.

"What's inflammation?" I hear you ask. Generally speaking, inflammation is a normal state for our bodies to be in, occasionally. This is called acute inflammation. When we have a cut or wound, the process of healing it is a type of inflammation that the body turns on when it needs to. Fevers are another type of acute inflammation that help the body get rid of the bacteria that have caused the cold or flu. Inflammation is led by cells and compounds that supercharge the immune system to help our bodies heal. When the situation is resolved, the immune system goes back to humming along in the background, getting rid of anything it feels could cause us trouble.

What does this have to do with periods? Well, our modern society has created a perfect recipe for chronic inflammation with the amount of stress we're under, how overfed yet undernourished we are, how much sugar we eat, and our lack of movement, sleep and emotional connection. This cocktail of factors keeps our immune systems overly active, fighting to get us back to our health status quo.

When we're in a state of chronic inflammation or slow, long-term inflammation that can last for prolonged periods of several months or even years,[10] this is bad news for our periods. Research tells us that inflammation can contribute to period pain, which I discuss in Chapter 8.

What does all of this mean for you? If you have a summer of boozing and lots of sugary treats, you could feel the impact on your periods in the autumn. That's wild, isn't it? Looking at it a bit differently, the changes that you make now will have the biggest impact on your period in three months' time, if not sooner!

Let's get into the nitty-gritty of what happens during menstruation.

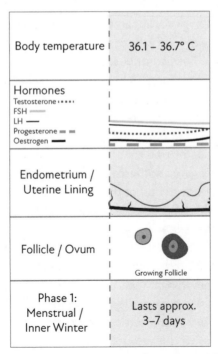

Body temperature	36.1 – 36.7° C
Hormones Testosterone ····· FSH —— LH —— Progesterone ▬ ▬ Oestrogen ▬	
Endometrium / Uterine Lining	
Follicle / Ovum	Growing Follicle
Phase 1: Menstrual / Inner Winter	Lasts approx. 3–7 days

An Overview of What's Happening During the Menstrual Phase

What's Happening Biologically?

Quite simply, menstruation happens when our oestrogen and progesterone drop low enough to signal to our bodies that it's time to shed the lining of the uterus, called the endometrium. This lining typically starts to rebuild toward the end of our periods, increasing in thickness during the follicular phase until the end of the menstrual cycle. If the mature egg that is released during ovulation isn't fertilized, the body knows it's time to restart the menstrual cycle by shedding the lining of the uterus so it has another opportunity to get us ready for ovulation.

The menstrual bleed flows from the uterus through the cervix and vagina to the vulva, where it is absorbed by whichever menstrual product we choose to use.

Did you know we're part of a select group of mammals that have a period? Most other mammals will reabsorb the uterine lining (this would be a great pub quiz question!). Human females have this cyclical process of building and shedding the lining of the uterus, which perhaps isn't that energy efficient, unlike most other biological processes in the body, yet still plays a key role in our health and fertility.

What's Happening Physically?

As we learned earlier in the chapter, there are many factors such as ovulation and chronic inflammation that can affect the quality and quantity of our periods. Just as we are all different from one another in all sorts of weird and wonderful ways, the flow of a normal period can vary hugely. Some of us can bleed lightly the first two days of our period, then heavy for two days, then light until the end. Some of us start off with light spotting, have a heavy flow and that's it. Some of us start our period, then stop for a day, then start again. Some of us can have lighter periods after we've given birth or come off hormonal contraception. Some of us can have fairly heavy bleeds for most of our menstrual years.

In a so-called normal period, the bleed can last from three to seven days and includes a mixture of blood, mucus, prostaglandins, tissue debris, cells from the lining of the vagina and bacteria from the vaginal microbiome.[11] The amount and colour of the blood can change each day of the period as the menstrual lining continues to shed and it makes its way down through the cervix and vagina.

The body will also release chemicals called anticoagulants that help thin the blood, preventing clots and helping blood from the lining of the uterus flow more easily.

What the Colour of Your Blood Means

Black	Old oxidized (exposed to oxygen) blood that wasn't pushed out of the uterus at the end of the last period, could indicate a vaginal blockage like a stuck tampon (go to your doctor ASAP if this the case!)
Brown	Beginning or end of period, old oxidized blood that wasn't pushed out of the uterus at end of the last period (this can be an indication of low progesterone – go to Chapter 6 for tips on supporting ovulation and progesterone production)
Dark red	Fresh menstrual blood
Bright red	Fresh menstrual blood (this is what we want!)
Pink	Can be an indicator of low oestrogen levels
Grey	Bacterial vaginosis – please see your doctor
Orange	Bacterial vaginosis or other infection – please see your doctor

How does your period compare? In the beginning, it might feel strange to think about focusing on the colour of our menstrual blood. I really encourage you to get comfortable with your menstrual blood. Doing this can help understand what's happening in our bodies and, crucially, if there's anything we need to address. I know not all of you are going to get on board with the idea of looking at your menstrual blood – some of you will want to simply get rid of or wash your menstrual products without looking at them (*never* flush menstrual products, by the way). Stay with me on this. Just take a peek and notice the colour. Then perhaps notice the consistency. Notice if you have a lot of large clots.

Some very small clots are normal, but it's the size and frequency of the clots that matter. If the blood clots are bigger than 2.5cm (a bit smaller than a £2 coin) and last throughout your period, that's a sign of a heavy period. I will talk more about heavy periods later in this chapter.

You may never be completely comfortable with your menstrual blood, and that's fine. But just being able to look at it will help you take notice of any issues that you may be having and start to connect the dots with your health.

What's Happening Hormonally?

Now let's look at what's happening hormonally during menstruation. When we don't fertilize the mature egg that gets released at ovulation, our body shifts out of conception-making (or trying to!) mode and our oestrogen and progesterone levels eventually drop to their lowest points right before, and in the first two days of, our periods.

Oestrogen is associated with conception and how the body tries to make this happen. Progesterone is the calming Mother Nature hormone that keeps you on an even keel. In her book, *How the Pill Changes Everything*, Dr Sarah Hill describes oestrogen as the hormone that's instrumental in getting our bodies ready for pregnancy each menstrual cycle.[12] It's also one of the hormones that guides the behaviours that put us in baby-making mode, i.e. suddenly finding your partner super attractive (more than you usually do!), or generally feeling much more playful and confident. Even if you're not trying to get pregnant, these hormones will have the same effects on mood and behaviours.

The drop in oestrogen and progesterone in the late luteal phase is what signals to our bodies that it's time to shed the lining of the uterus. It also signals to the body that it's time to stimulate the release of prostaglandins, the hormone-like compounds that help the blood flow down the uterus.

Prostaglandins have a bad rap because we associate them with premenstrual and period pain (see Chapter 8). Prostaglandins also help trigger the shedding of the lining of the uterus, otherwise known as the endometrium, by restricting the oxygen supply in the cells of the womb lining. These cells die and this is what is shed during menstruation. Prostaglandins also trigger uterine muscle contractions, which push the endometrium out of the uterus and cervix to the vagina and vulva.

OESTRADIOL

During our menstruating years, when we talk about oestrogen, we're typically talking about oestradiol, the primary form of oestrogen that is produced by the ovaries during this time. There are three other forms of oestrogen to be aware of: oestrone, which is produced by the adrenal glands (two tiny tissues that sit on top of the kidneys) and is the predominant form of oestrogen during the menopause and post-menopausal years. Many women think that oestrogen production fully shuts down after menopause and that's simply not true. We just produce less, and a less powerful form.

The other two are forms of oestrogen that are produced primarily during pregnancy: oestriol and oestetrol. Oestriol is produced by the placenta and oestetrol is produced by the fetus' liver.

In this book, when I talk about oestrogen, I'm typically referring to oestradiol, unless I say otherwise.

Think back to how you might feel on days 1 and 2 of your period. The words I usually hear about this time in our menstrual cycles are: flat, tired, apathetic, effortful. And do you notice that around the halfway mark of your period, you feel like you've got a bit of a kick-start? That's because of follicle stimulating hormone (FSH), which does what it says on the tin: it stimulates the follicles in our ovaries to start the nearly year-long process of growing a primordial follicle into the mature egg that is released during ovulation. FSH typically starts to rise a few days before the end of our last menstrual cycle.[13] It then activates the aromatase enzyme in the granulosa cells in our ovaries, which then initiates the gradual rise in oestrogen after our periods start.[14]

This is why many of us have that "out of the woods" feeling around day 3 or 4 of menstruation and just simply start to feel a bit like ourselves again. This rising oestrogen also starts to stimulate the regrowth of the lining of the uterus.[15] Basically, while we have our periods, we're also beginning to regrow the endometrial lining that will be shed during our next period – how amazing are our bodies?

We have oestrogen receptors all over our bodies and the oestrogen that's produced from our ovaries acts like a key that opens up the locked receptors. Think back to Chapter 2, where I talked about hormones and this idea of a lock (the hormone receptor) and key (the hormone). Hormones guide hundreds of functions in the body, including our energy, mood and behaviour. At the beginning of our periods, our oestrogen levels are low, and this can have an impact on our behaviour, mood, emotions and thoughts.

Oestrogen is generally associated with conception (and we'll get into the detail of how it drives this in the next chapter), but that's not all this powerful hormone is good for. Here's a list of oestrogen influences:[16, 17]

- Metabolism (how quickly and how well you digest and break down food, how quickly digestion turns into bowel

movements and how effectively we break down proteins in the liver)
- How we store fat (the rise of oestrogen after puberty is typically associated with the development of breasts and curves around the hips and tummy)
- Vaginal lubrication and thickness of vaginal wall
- The thickening of the lining of the uterus
- The growth of the egg follicle
- Immune function
- Brain function
- Sodium levels and water retention
- Pain transmission
- Bone health
- Blood vessel function
- Blood clotting
- Cholesterol levels, increasing HDL (the protective form of cholesterol) and decreasing LDL (the damaging form of cholesterol) cholesterol
- Mental health and cognition

Oestradiol is created from cholesterol in the ovaries. We need dietary cholesterol to make cholesterol in the body, which is then converted into hormones like oestradiol. Forget what you've heard about no-fat or low-fat diets. We need to eat fat to make hormones like oestrogen and progesterone!

What Are the Mental and Social Effects of the Menstrual Phase?

Remember the idea of using the seasons to connect with each phase of our menstrual cycle that we discussed in Chapter 2? Based on how we feel during our period, it seems fitting to call this the winter of our menstrual cycles.

Lower levels of oestrogen can affect our emotional wellbeing and mental state. Take its effect on serotonin, the chemical that functions both as a neurotransmitter and a hormone, for example. Serotonin is known as our happy hormone. Oestrogen is thought to be connected to the serotonergic system[18] (the system that makes serotonin), with oestrogen and serotonin receptors coexisting in a wide variety of cells in a number of different tissues in the body. Some animal studies have shown that oestradiol increases the production of tryptophan,[19] an amino acid that is required for serotonin production. Oestradiol has been connected with increased serotonin levels, which means that as our oestrogen levels rise, so does our ability to make serotonin.[20] Conversely, when oestrogen levels are low, our serotonin levels are also low, which can have a negative effect on our moods, especially in the first two to three days of our period.

This can give us a helpful framework for thinking about our moods and our emotional wellbeing during our periods.

In this phase, we're shedding what doesn't serve us anymore and making space for something new. This process is not only physical; it can be mental and emotional too.

Think about how you feel during your period. Do you feel as though you want to turn inward? Perhaps this is when you become more reflective and evaluate certain events and situations in your life.

In their book, *Wild Power*, Alexandra Pope and Sjanie Hugo Wurlitzer describe menstruation as "the engine room of your power ... the prime time to plant the seeds of your intentions for the coming cycle and beyond."[21]

If we are to truly use menstruation as a time to think of the future and plant intentions, we must allow ourselves time and space to slow down. And that can be hard, can't it? Most of us live lives that don't give us a lot of time to take our foot off the accelerator, even a little bit. But I bet, if you really looked, you could find a way to introduce a little slowness into the days you have your period. Small tweaks can make all the difference.

Could you try some of the following small tweaks?

- Make an effort to be at home the evenings you have your period, especially the first two days
- Take a proper lunch break
- Phone (don't text!) a friend for a nice slow chat (remind yourself of all the time you used to spend talking on the phone when you were a teenager), or even go old school and write a letter (or postcard!)
- Spend time journalling. If you find journalling challenging, try using prompts to help focus your thinking or write a few words that resonate
- Get up a little earlier so you can have some quiet time before the rest of your house wakes up
- Stare out of the window instead of being on your phone on your train or tube journey home. *Niksen*, a Dutch word for doing absolutely nothing or being idle, says that purposeless activities like just hanging out and listening to music are helpful for encouraging us to just be. Remember: we're human **BE**ings, not human **DO**ings, and this time just doing nothing is an opportunity to rest

There is some research that tells us that the low oestrogen in this phase can have several effects on our mental abilities, although these studies are not always entirely conclusive and some of the findings contradict each other. What we know is that oestrogen (and progesterone) interacts with the neurotransmitter systems that are associated with cognition, executive function, learning and memory: those of serotonin, GABA, acetylcholine, dopamine and glutamine.[22]
  We might find that during our periods:

- Our memories may not be as strong[23]
- We might struggle to concentrate
- We might be more inwardly focused
- Our motivation might be lower
- Tasks involving visualization and spatial abilities might be easier[24]

It's really important to add the caveat that none of this is inevitable and will be affected by your individual circumstances. However, it can be helpful to be aware of these changes if you find that you're a little forgetful or that you must work harder to focus during your period.

Anecdotal evidence tells us that menstruation is the time where our abilities of evaluation and analysis will be at their strongest. This is the time when we may find a greater connection with our inner wisdom and intuition. Slowing down gives us the space to take stock and look at where we are in our lives. And this doesn't necessarily mean you have to do a wholesale review of everything that's happening in your life. It doesn't have to get that deep. You might reflect on a particular situation or moment and give yourself the time to really think through it.

Good things to schedule for this time:

- Prepare for a chat with a mentor or for an appraisal at work. This might feel counterintuitive, but this is also a time where if we slow down, we can give ourselves the opportunity to see how we really feel about a particular work situation
- Review your goals from the last year / quarter / month and set some new short-term goals
- A long journalling session, guided or not, in which you give yourself space to leave everything on the page
- A session of yoga nidra, or yogic sleep, to give your brain a bit of a chance to rest

From a social perspective, you might find that part of this feeling of turning inward includes a feeling of wanting to withdraw from social settings that you'd normally be up for. If you think about what's happening physically and the act of shedding that's happening inside your uterus, it makes sense that emotionally, we might switch into hibernation mode. I know we're not bears hunkering down for a long winter, but if this is the winter of our menstrual cycles, you may notice that you feel a physical longing to be closer to home and what's comfortable.

What's Normal During Your Period?

So, what's normal? When I talk about what's normal in each phase of the menstrual cycle in this book, this isn't what we've accepted as *culturally* normal. As I noted earlier, for a number of reasons we've accepted a cultural narrative that periods are supposed to be, quite frankly, really shitty. We've accepted that we're supposed to dread our periods or, at the very least, feel pretty rubbish for a few days each month.

In this section, what I'll be describing as normal is what is *biologically and physically* normal for someone who has a period each cycle. You may experience some or all of them. Use the tools in this chapter to figure out what your normal is and remind yourself that severe pain, exhaustion and very heavy bleeding are not normal.

Here's how we would define a physically normal period:

A normal period is losing up to 60ml (the average is about 30ml),[25] having bright red blood for the majority of the time, very little pain, perhaps some light cramping or aches, slightly lower energy levels, a menstrual flow that slows down or doesn't get heavier at night and lasts no longer than seven days. Interestingly, research was done on menstruating female astronauts in space, who were originally thought to have retrograde menstruation due to zero gravity. Basically, it was assumed that menstrual blood and fluid would reverse itself, flowing back into the womb. It was found that menstruation continues as normal, due to prostaglandins that stimulate the uterine contractions that push the menstrual fluid out of the womb. Gravity has no effect on these contractions.[26, 27]

If you're wondering how much blood you actually lose, here's a way to work it out:

- Regular tampons and pads hold about 5ml of fluid, fully soaked
- Super tampons and pads hold about 10ml of fluid, fully soaked
- Depending on the brand, menstrual cups can hold 15–60ml at a time
- Depending on the brand and level of absorbency, period underwear can hold 25–45ml of fluid, fully soaked

Here are some physical signs that are completely normal during this phase:

- Lower energy
- Slight discomfort
- Appetite changes
- Slightly flat mood, perhaps affected by lower energy
- Feeling a bit more reflective
- Feeling a little less social

All of this is okay and is a sign from our bodies telling us to slow down and nurture ourselves a little bit more than we would usually do.

With everything the body is doing, it makes sense that we'll feel a little less energetic. For example, I've really noticed that on days 1 and 2, my energy is at its lowest point. My instinct is to push through and keep running around the way I usually do. I now know that it's better for me to slow down and allow myself extra time to do things. I do my best to avoid rushing from place to place and appointment to appointment (which is my modus operandi!), minimize the work I do in the evenings and take the time to take care of myself.

We're also slightly insulin-resistant during our period (and just before) due to low oestrogen[28] and progesterone. This can have an impact on our energy levels because our body must work harder to use the sugar from the carbohydrates we've eaten. A 2010 study that followed 257 healthy, regularly menstruating women for two menstrual cycles found that both oestrogen and progesterone increase insulin sensitivity, which means that it's easier for insulin from our pancreas to help sugar (which comes from our digestive system breaking down the carbohydrates we've eaten) move through the blood and into our cells. The participants in this study had higher insulin sensitivity during the follicular, ovulatory and early luteal phases, when oestrogen and progesterone levels were higher. During their late luteal and menstrual phases, they were more insulin-resistant due to lower levels of oestrogen and progesterone.[29] What does this mean for you in practice? Be kind to yourself and know that it's normal to have lower energy during and before your period. Nourish your body with foods that support your energy levels. Go back to the Balanced Plate (page 38) if you need a little refresher. If you notice your energy flagging, start to explore what's happening and where the energy drains are coming from. Are you getting enough sleep? Are you taking breaks during the day? Do you have energy vampires in your life that take without giving anything back?

Self-care is a huge buzzword right now, so you might be nodding your head at the idea of slowing down during your period (or maybe you're resisting it! Dig a little deeper and ask yourself why you're resisting the idea of slowing down). What I've seen in my clinical practice is that when my clients allow themselves to move at a slightly slower pace and take a little more time during their period, it has a positive effect on their energy levels during the rest of their menstrual cycle.

I know it's hard. We're living in a time where hustle culture is put on a pedestal and society values people who never stop working. In yoga philosophy, there's the concept of masculine and feminine energy, or shiva and shakti. Masculine energy, symbolized by the sun, is pervasive in

Western culture. It's the 24/7 hustle, I'll sleep when I'm dead mindset. Feminine energy, symbolized by the moon, aligns with our menstrual cycles, recognizes that there's a time to work hard and equally recognizes the restorative value of rest and recovery.

If slowing all the way down during your period seems too hard, ask yourself what you could do to slow down to 95 per cent of your capacity, rather than 100 per cent.

What's Not Normal During Your Period?
There are a few things to watch out for that aren't normal.

- A very light period that lasts less than three days
- A light period that lasts for two weeks
- A heavy period that lasts longer than seven days (the medical term for this is menorrhagia)
- Losing more than 80ml of menstrual blood per cycle
- A period where you're changing your pad / tampon / cup every one to two hours or more (this is called flooding), and you're constantly worried about blood soaking through to your clothes
- Painful periods (dysmenorrhea)
- Feeling exhausted throughout your entire period
- A bleed that is very light red, black, grey, excessively brown or pink in colour
- Large clots
- Headaches / migraines
- Nausea
- Mood swings
- Complete loss of appetite

These are all signs that there is something wrong and needs to be investigated.

Many of the issues I see around periods are typically related to too much inflammation in the body, which can increase period pain. For a refresher on inflammation, see page 65.

It's when the inflammation never stops that we can run into health problems, such as the pain that more and more women are experiencing with their periods. I talk about period pain more extensively in Chapter 8.

Nutrient deficiencies, hormonal imbalances and other conditions such as fibroids, endometriosis and an underactive or overactive thyroid can also contribute to period problems.

Eloise's Story

Eloise came to me because of really painful periods due to endometriosis. She had had a laparoscopy, a keyhole surgery that is used to diagnose endometriosis. Eloise's surgeons were also able to remove most of the endometrial tissue from the outside of her uterus, bowels and rectum during the surgery. Post-surgery, Eloise was keen to make sure she was doing everything she could to prevent the return of her most debilitating endometriosis symptoms: the period pain and bloating.

We spent a lot of time looking at what we could do to support her immune system to reduce inflammation and support her gut health. We started by looking at what Eloise was eating and building a plan that would address the habits that were contributing to the painful periods and digestive issues that often found her running to the loo or having trouble zipping up her jeans.

After years of working at a highly stressful job, Eloise had a habit of relaxing at the end of the day with a bag of Haribo and a large glass (or two, or three ...) of red wine. She admitted that she would find her sugar habit the hardest thing to break because she really looked forward to her sweet treat at the end of each day. I asked her to notice how she felt before, during and after she ate the Haribo. She said that she looked forward to snacking on her favourite treats and loved the taste of them, but when she was finished, she always felt guilty, tired and a bit remorseful.

To make sure she wasn't overwhelmed, we started by looking at what she could do to replace the Haribo habit with something that still gave her that hit of sweetness and helped her relax. I asked her to start buying green grapes, pineapple and mango, and eat those alongside the Haribo. I also asked Eloise to make a list of things she found relaxing, and choose one of those things to do as well.

Eventually, Eloise found a new evening habit of eating fruit salad and reading a good book that she looked forward to as much as snacking on Haribo. After we replaced this habit, we looked at her daily wine habit. Eloise had got into the practice of drinking lots of coffee throughout the day to keep her going and then using wine to unwind at night. We explored the emotions around her nightly glass of wine, and I asked her to consider replacing wine with herbal tea. She laughed and said that herbal tea wouldn't touch the sides, so I asked her to start by only drinking on alternate nights during the week and limit herself to two drinks on Friday and Saturday night instead.

All of the alcohol and sugar Eloise was eating and drinking was contributing to the inflammation that increased the pain with her periods. My priority in working with her was looking at how we could reduce inflammation. Reducing sugar and alcohol was the obvious first step for me, so we had to change the habits she had created around these areas, but she also had to feel that we weren't just cutting things out that she enjoyed. We worked together to find some fun new recipes for her to try and this helped to get her excited about cooking again. This also helped to boost Eloise's vegetable and fruit intake to at least ten portions a day: seven mainly green, leafy vegetables and three pieces of fruit. Finally, we also looked at her gut health to make sure her gut microbiome was robust enough to help break down the excess oestrogen that was in her system and stop her cycling between constipation and diarrhoea.

After 12 weeks, Eloise said that she had completely broken her sugar and wine habits and was really enjoying exploring different ways of adding vegetables into her daily meals. She reported that her digestive system had settled down and that her periods weren't nearly as painful as they used to be.

Improving Your Period with Food

During your period, it's natural to have a bit less energy and to feel a few aches and twinges. Optimizing your nutrition is an effective way of boosting energy levels, improving mood and reducing pain and cramps. I'll be talking a lot about what we can add in (not just depriving you of your favourite stuff!) and breaking down the key nutrients that are needed for healthy periods.

In my clinical practice, I always start clients off by looking at what they can *add* before we even think about taking anything away. Once they've successfully added new foods in, I then look at what they're eating and drinking that isn't working for them.

Sugar and alcohol are two of the biggest culprits of inflammation and can exacerbate painful periods. I would really encourage you to look, honestly, at how much sugar you eat each day and how often you drink alcohol.

I'm not one for demonizing food groups, but many of us can find ourselves drinking a little too often or relying on alcohol to relax, which can play havoc with our hormones, as I discussed in Chapter 3.

If you choose to drink, ideally you're drinking one to two glasses of alcohol, twice a week, maximum. If you choose to eat sugary foods, then it's looking at how often you're having sweets. You don't need to have something sweet to end each meal. We'd all benefit from going back to seeing sugary food as an occasional extra, not a daily necessity.

Let's look at the key nutrients and foods for healthy periods. All the foods in this section are even more beneficial during this phase of your menstrual cycle. However, you do not need to limit them to this time, as they will be helpful all throughout your cycle, incorporated as part of the Balanced Plate I went through on page 38.

KEY NUTRIENTS AND FOODS FOR THE MENSTRUAL PHASE

Iron: heme: grass-fed beef and lamb, dark poultry meat
Iron: non-heme: chickpeas/garbanzo beans, lentils, quinoa, kidney beans, kale
Vitamin C: citrus, kiwi, strawberries, raspberries, blueberries, broccoli, red pepper, yellow pepper
Copper: organic beef liver, oyster, potatoes, mushrooms, cashews, crab, sunflower seeds, dark / bittersweet chocolate
Magnesium: leafy green vegetables (like kale, rocket/ arugula, watercress and spinach), nuts and seeds
Vitamin A: organic beef liver, carrots, pumpkin, sweet potato, spinach, cod liver oil, spring/collard greens, kale
Vitamin B12: organic red meat, dairy and eggs
Omega-3: oily fish (SMASHHT: salmon, mackerel, anchovies, sardines, haddock, herring, trout), algae
Vitamin K: natto (fermented soybeans), chard, organic beef or chicken liver, spring/collard greens, spinach, kale, broccoli

Iron and Vitamin C (and Copper!)

Iron plays an important role in energy production, transporting oxygen through the blood and blood rebuilding, which is important during menstruation, as we can lose anywhere between 30 and 80ml of menstrual blood, depending on how heavy our periods are.

Iron loss due to menstruation is the most frequent cause of iron deficiency anaemia among women of reproductive age. A 2019 Italian study found that women with heavy periods lose five to six times more iron per cycle than women with healthy periods who lose, on average, 1mg of iron per cycle.[30] Iron is important for making red blood cells, and if there isn't enough iron or the body is not able to use iron effectively, this can lead to iron deficiency anaemia. The symptoms of iron deficiency anaemia[31] are:

- Continual feeling of low energy
- Low moods
- Menstrual headaches and migraines
- Lethargy
- Breathlessness
- Heavy periods
- Spoon-shaped nails
- Weak nails
- Very pale skin
- Hair loss
- White marks in nail beds

Eating iron-rich foods helps the body generate new blood and replace what has been lost during menstruation. According to the NHS, those of us that menstruate need about 14.8mg of iron each day,[32] which can come from food or supplements. As many of us shift toward vegetarianism and veganism, I'm starting to see more cases of low iron and iron deficiency anaemia in clinic. These women are enthusiastic about changing the way they eat for health, religious or ethical reasons, but they aren't necessarily eating enough of the plant-based iron foods that will give them energy and support healthy menstruation. It's not all bad news: if you're vegetarian or vegan, please be intentional about including enough iron, vitamin C and copper foods in your meals each day. There's no reason why you can't get enough of these essential nutrients in your meals with a well-planned approach.

Copper is often left out of discussions about iron, but this mineral is important for making sure our bodies are able to effectively use the iron we get from food and supplements, as well as the iron that we store (this is called ferritin). When our body's iron stores are too low, copper gets redistributed to tissues that are key for regulating iron balance, including the blood.[33] If you are anaemic and taking iron supplements, it's important that you have sources of copper in your diet, as too much iron can be inflammatory and can deplete copper. We need about 900mcg (micrograms, not mg!) of copper each day, which can be obtained through a variety of plant and animal foods.[34]

When it comes to iron from foods, there are two types we need to consider: heme and non-heme iron.

Heme iron, which typically comes from animal products such as grass-fed beef and lamb, is easier for the body to absorb and then use. About 40 per cent of this type of iron is absorbed by the body.[35]

Non-heme iron, which comes from plant-based sources, is less able to be used by the body. So if you're a vegan or vegetarian, or even just flirting with eating less meat, you'll need to eat a lot more non-heme iron foods, such as chickpeas/garbanzo beans, lentils, quinoa, kidney beans and kale – and, crucially, they need to be paired with vitamin C foods. Eating vitamin C with a meal can greatly increase non-heme iron absorption, so squeeze lemon over your quinoa salad or have broccoli with your lentils!

Example Sources of Heme Iron[36]	Milligrams
100g / 3½oz grass-fed organic minced / ground beef	2.6
100g / 3½oz grass-fed ribeye	2.2
28g / 1oz lamb's liver	2.1
100g / 3½oz minced / ground lamb	1.6
28g / 1oz beef liver	1.4

Example Sources of Non-heme Iron[37]	Milligrams
200g / 7oz cooked lentils	8.8
150g / 5½oz cooked kidney beans	5.2
140g / 5oz cooked chickpeas/garbanzo beans	4.7
150g / 5½oz dried black beans	3.3
185g / 6½oz cooked quinoa	2.8
2 tbsp tahini	2.7
100g / 3½oz Swiss chard	1.8
100g / 3½oz mustard greens	1.6

Example Sources of Vitamin C[38]	Milligrams
100g / 3½oz raw kale	93.4
91g / 3oz raw broccoli	81.2
1 medium orange	63.4
28g / 1oz / ¼ cup blueberries	2.7
1 lemon wedge	2.6

Example Sources of Copper[39]	Milligrams
68g / 2½oz (1 slice) organic beef liver	9.72
100g / 3½oz dried shiitake mushrooms	5.2
6 oysters	3.8
245g / 9oz / 1 cup mashed sweet potatoes	0.7
28g / 1oz / ¼ cup cashews	0.6
1 square dark / bittersweet chocolate	0.5

Magnesium

Magnesium is another important nutrient for better periods.

It is used in over 300 functions in the body, including the way we make energy, the way our brain functions, our digestive system, as well as our heart and bone health. Over-farming the soil means that we're not getting as much magnesium from our food as we did in the past.[40] Chronic stress can also increase magnesium deficiency because of the nutrient's role in calming the nervous system. This creates a vicious cycle of chronic stress, further magnesium depletion, which reduces our resilience and ability to bounce back from stressful situations.

The signs and symptoms of magnesium deficiency[41] are:

- Eye twitches
- Fatigue
- Low moods / apathy
- Muscle weakness
- Chocolate cravings
- Muscle cramps and twitches
- Headaches / migraines
- Low bone mineral density / osteoporosis
- High blood pressure

Magnesium is nature's relaxing mineral, which means that when it comes to periods, it's fantastic for balancing the low moods that some of us may experience.

Most of us think about magnesium as a way of soothing tense muscles after a long gym session – think Epsom salts baths. Magnesium can also be hugely beneficial for easing period cramps and pain. The muscular lining of the uterus contracts when we have our periods to help the blood flow down. If we have too much inflammation, these contractions can be painful, as I discuss further in Chapter 8. Magnesium is a powerful anti-inflammatory mineral that can help manage contractions by relaxing the muscles. Adding a daily magnesium supplement is a great way to reduce chronic inflammation on an ongoing basis.

For those of us who get menstrual headaches and migraines, magnesium is a fantastic way to give yourself a bit of short-term relief.

On average, menstruating women need about 300mg of magnesium each day, or more if you're under a significant amount of stress. If you're nodding along, thinking about how stressed you feel, it's worth adding magnesium to your daily supplement routine. Magnesium is one of my favourite all-round supplements. It's great for calming nervous energy, relaxing sore muscles, balancing blood sugar levels and reducing premenstrual food cravings, but sadly many of us are deficient.[42] In times of significant stress, I will typically recommend that my clients take at least 240mg of magnesium glycinate each day, alongside what they get through food.

And of course, there are great ways to get magnesium in your meals. Leafy green vegetables like kale, rocket/arugula, watercress and spinach are a great option. If you're not up for more vegetables, pumpkin seeds and almonds also have a lot of magnesium, so spread some almond butter on some sliced banana for a sweet treat during your period!

Example Sources of Magnesium[43]	Milligrams
28g / 1oz / 3 tbsp pumpkin seeds	150
28g / 1oz / ¼ cup cashews	82
28g / 1oz dark / bittersweet chocolate	64
1 medium avocado	58
100g / 3½oz uncooked kale	34

Vitamin A

Did your parents ever tell you that eating your carrots would help you see better in the dark? That's the power of carotenoids, one of the two forms of vitamin A, which comes from plants such as squash, sweet potatoes, pumpkins, spinach and kale. The other type, preformed vitamin A, comes from animal sources like beef liver, cod liver, tuna, eggs, butter and milk. Aside from its eye-health-boosting benefits, vitamin A is important for blood building and ensuring we have enough haemoglobin, the protein that transports oxygen through our blood.[44] Vitamin A also plays well with iron and copper to help make red blood cells, which is important, especially during our periods, when we lose blood through our menstrual fluid.

Some limited research suggests that vitamin A deficiency may be a contributing factor in heavy periods. Anecdotally, we can link vitamin A with the thyroid, as we need it to regulate thyroid hormone metabolism. Heavy periods are a symptom of an underactive thyroid, or hypothyroidism. This is another example of how interconnected our bodies are: a deficiency of a single vitamin can affect other parts of the body.

We must be careful when supplementing vitamin A. Along with D, E and K, it's a fat-soluble vitamin, which means that we store any excess in our fat tissue and liver, rather than excreting it through our urine like other vitamins. With this Goldilocks vitamin, focus on getting enough through food rather than only through supplementation.

Similarly to iron, with its two forms, heme and non-heme, plant-based vitamin A is less easily absorbed and gets converted into retinol in the small intestine. Preformed vitamin A from animal sources converts easily into retinol. We need about 700mcg (micrograms) RAE (retinol activity equivalents) from different types of vitamin A each day.[45] A small note: if you are trying to conceive, please avoid high-dose preformed vitamin A supplementation, as it can have a negative effect on the development of the embryo.[46] Instead, continue to include a wide range of vitamin A foods in your meals each day.

Example Sources of Vitamin A[47]	Micrograms RAE (retinol activity equivalents)
85g / 3oz beef liver	6582
1 baked sweet potato	1400
1 tsp cod liver oil	1350
45g / 1½oz cooked spinach	573
1 cooked carrot	392
100g / 3½oz cooked spring/collard greens	380
100g / 3½oz cooked kale	146

Vitamin B12

Vitamin B12, like iron, is another nutrient that's important for making red blood cells, which means that it's necessary for healthy periods. It's also needed for our body to make energy, for nervous system support and to support our moods.

Vitamin B12 is a water-soluble vitamin, so we need to regularly replenish our levels through food and supplements because we cannot store extra amounts. When we have too much in our body, it gets passed through our urine.

The signs and symptoms of vitamin B12 deficiency[48] are:

- Fatigue and weakness
- Numbness and tingling of the hands and feet
- Memory loss
- Disorientation and balance issues
- Appetite loss
- Sore tongue
- Constipation
- Depression
- Pale skin
- Breathlessness
- Heart palpitations
- Tinnitus
- Mouth ulcers

It's easy to get all the vitamin B12 you need each day (we need about 2.4mcg each day)[49] if high-quality meat, dairy and seafood are included in your meals. Unless they eat a well-planned diet, it can be harder for vegans to get enough vitamin B12. Nutritional yeast is great (some brands have between 2 to 5mcg of vitamin B12 per tablespoon), but do you want to eat it every day? If you do, then great! I always recommend that vegan clients take a vitamin B12 supplement or a multivitamin that contains high-quality B12, such as methylcobalamin.

Example Sources of Vitamin B12[50]	Micrograms
28g / 1oz beef liver	19.8
65g / 2¼oz herring	12.2
100g / 3½oz wild Alaskan salmon	7.8
1 egg	3.8
100g / 3½oz lamb shoulder	3.1

Omega-3 Fatty Acids

Omega-3 fatty acids are a type of fat that we must get from food because we cannot make them ourselves. They are highly anti-inflammatory, so foods containing these fatty acids are helpful for managing mood changes, period pain and reducing headaches, migraines and acne. For painful periods, consistently adding these fatty acids into your meals can help reduce excess prostaglandins, the hormone-like compounds that can increase period pain. If you don't fancy eating these foods, an omega-3 fish oil or algae capsule is a great addition into a daily supplement regime.

Some research backs the use of omega-3 fatty acids to reduce period pain. One research study conducted with a small group of young women found that the intensity of their period pain was reduced after taking omega-3 capsules daily for three months,[51] while another study that compared usage of fish oil with ibuprofen for period pain found that those that were taking omega-3 capsules experienced a greater reduction in their pain levels.[52] Sounds good, doesn't it?

Some organizations suggest we should consume around 1.1g of omega-3 fatty acids each day,[53] with an equal amount of DHA and EPA. When I talk about these fats with my clients, I always discuss the double-edged sword of eating fish. On one hand, oily fish is a brilliant source of omega-3 fatty acids, and a great source of protein, vitamin B12 and zinc. On the other hand, we must consider the environment the fish comes from. Our oceans and lakes are becoming polluted with microplastics and different forms of waste, which we ingest when we eat food from these places – doesn't sound very appetizing, does it?

With this in mind, I recommend that you eat seafood a maximum of three times per week. Here's a fun acronym to help remind you of the best types of oily fish:

S – sardines
M – mackerel
A – anchovies
S – salmon
H – herring
H – haddock
T – trout

For vegetarians and vegans, algae is the best source of omega-3 compared to flaxseed because it converts more easily from alpha-linolenic acid (ALA) to omega-3 fatty acid than flaxseed.

Example Sources of Omega-3 Fatty Acids[54]	Milligrams
100g / 3½oz wild Atlantic mackerel	2670
100g / 3½oz kippered herring	2365
100g / 3½oz wild Alaskan salmon	2018
5 anchovies	423
2 sardines	355

Vitamin K

Like iron and vitamin A, there are two types of vitamin K: K1 and K2. If you struggle with heavy periods, this is a helpful vitamin to add into your meals. Vitamin K is required by the body for regulation of blood clotting, so when we're even slightly deficient, this can contribute to heavy periods[55] (along with an imbalance between oestrogen and progesterone, the primary reason for heavy menstrual bleeding). True deficiency is exceedingly rare because vitamin K is another fat-soluble vitamin, so we can store it in our fat tissue.

Vitamin K1, made by plants, typically from dark leafy greens, is the primary form of vitamin K that many of us get in our diets. The other form of vitamin K, K2, is made from the microbiome in our gut, and is also found in fermented foods like natto (a Japanese fermented soybean dish) and sauerkraut, as well as some animal products like liver and egg yolks. We need about 90mcg (micrograms) per day.[56]

Example Sources of Vitamin K2[57]	Micrograms
25g / 1oz natto	275.85
50g / 1¾oz organic beef liver	53
2 egg yolks	31
25g / 1oz butter	5.25

Example Sources of Vitamin K1	
100g / 3½oz Swiss chard	830
100g / 3½oz raw kale	389
100g / 3½oz cooked broccoli	141

Recipes for the Menstrual Phase

On the next two pages I've included a couple of my favourite recipes for the menstrual phase. I hope you enjoy them!

'KALE CRISPS

Prep and cook time: 30 minutes
Serves: 1–2

What you need:

200g / 7oz curly green or purple kale
15–30ml / ½–1fl oz olive oil
Seasonings of choice (such as a pinch of sea salt with 1 tsp of
    any of the following: cumin powder, chilli powder, rosemary
    or za'atar)

How to make it:

1. Preheat the oven to 100°C fan / 120°C / 250°F /
   gas mark 1. Rinse and dry the kale leaves with paper
   towels, then tear into smaller pieces, putting the
   large stems aside for smoothies or stocks.
2. Put the kale pieces into a large mixing bowl
   and drizzle with the olive oil. Use your hands to
   massage the oil into the kale and then add your
   choice of seasonings, making sure everything is
   evenly coated.
3. Spread the kale pieces over two large baking
   sheets, ensuring the leaves overlap as little as
   possible, so they get crisp.
4. Bake for 20–25 minutes or until the kale is crispy.
   Keep your eye on it close to the end of the cooking
   time because the kale can burn easily if the oven is
   too hot.
5. Remove from the oven and let cool slightly – the
   chips will crisp up even more once out of the oven.
6. Enjoy!

BERRY BLITZ

Prep and cook time: 5 minutes
Serves: 1

What you need:

65g / 2¼oz / ½ cup mixed berries (you can use fresh or frozen)
1 tsp ground cinnamon, plus extra for dusting
2 handfuls frozen kale
½ avocado
1 tbsp sunflower seeds
1 heaped tbsp almond butter
1–2 tbsp organic Greek yogurt
200ml / 7fl oz / 1 scant cup almond milk

How to make it:

1. Put all the ingredients into a blender.
2. Blend for 30–60 seconds, depending on your preferred thickness.
3. Pour into a glass, garnish with a dusting of cinnamon and enjoy!

Improving Your Period With Exercise and Movement

This is the time in your menstrual cycle where it's nice to shift toward lower impact exercise, especially during the first two days of your period. This is when your energy levels are likely to be at their lowest, due to low levels of oestrogen.

I know some of you are keen on getting your daily workout in no matter what, so planning your exercise around your menstrual cycle might be a new idea. Hear me out.

A 2016 study showed that 41.7 per cent of exercising women in the UK believe that their menstrual cycle has a negative impact on exercise training and performance.[58] I'd love to help all of us understand that this doesn't have to be the case. It's so important for us to listen to our bodies and give them what they need. That includes the right exercise and physical movement for how we feel during each phase of our menstrual cycle. We've been conditioned to power through when we're not feeling great and I invite you to think about how you can flip this idea on its head.

If you find that your energy levels are good during your period and you want to move, I encourage you to avoid going at your maximum capacity and, crucially, accept that you won't be able to go all out. Equally, if you've tuned into your body and find yourself wanting to move a little slower or not at all, then I urge you to listen.

For those of you who want to continue moving your body during your period, try gentle exercise such as restorative or slow flow yoga, walking and swimming, especially during the first few days.

Go slowly, listen to your body and give yourself what you need during this time. If you're twitching reading this, thinking, "How the hell am I going to slow down?", pushing yourself during your period can have negative effects on your performance throughout the rest of your menstrual cycle. Low oestrogen levels during menstruation mean that we're more prone to soft tissue injuries because of oestrogen's effect on increasing collagen in connective tissue. A small study of 38 female athletes over three years found that a significant number of ACL (anterior cruciate ligament) or knee injuries occurred on day 1 and 2 of menstruation.[59] If you're still skeptical, try a little experiment. During your next period, reduce your exercise time by 20 per cent and see how it affects your performance during the rest of your menstrual cycle.

A Few Yoga Poses for When You're on Your Period

Cobbler's pose / *Baddha Konasana*

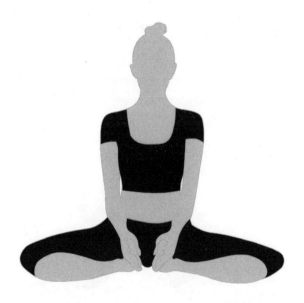

This pose helps open up the pelvis to support healthy blood flow around the uterus, supports the hips and creates lightness. *Baddha konasana* can be really helpful for painful periods, especially for those with endometriosis and adenomyosis, where the instinct may be to curl up in a ball and remain stationary as a way of reducing the pain.

Yogi's squat / *Malasana*

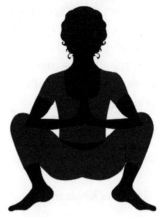

This is another pelvic and hip opener that can relieve the heaviness that many of us may feel on day 1 or 2 of our periods. While doing the pose, it's important to lift and squeeze the pelvic floor to connect with the abdominal muscles. This will help keep the chest and head lifted and open the hips even further.

Cat-cow pose / *Bitilasana Marjaryasana*

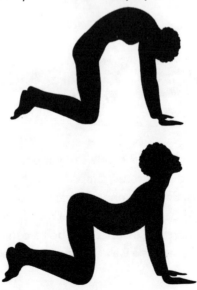

Cat-cow is a lovely way to add some gentle pelvic movement during menstruation. Start from the pelvis, tilting it upward, and imagine yourself like a wave rippling forward toward your head. Move into cat pose by tipping the pelvis downward, doming the shoulders and bringing the chin toward the chest.

BOX BREATHING

Here's a lovely breathing technique for those of you who are visual. Box breathing (also known as tactical breathing) offers the image of a box to help guide the breath.

Breathing is great to calm the nervous system, reduce anxiety and manage pain, which can be heightened during our periods.

Here's how to do it: take a long, slow breath in for four counts through your nose. Hold for four counts. Exhale for four long, slow counts through your nose. Hold for four counts. As you do this breathing exercise, visualize drawing a box as you go through each step. Do this as many times as you need!

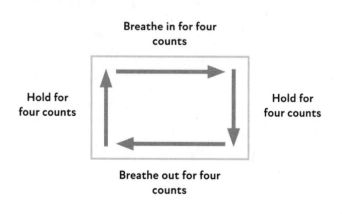

Breathe in for four counts

Hold for four counts

Hold for four counts

Breathe out for four counts

What You Can Try During the Menstrual Phase

Here's a summary of the recommendations in this chapter. Don't feel you have to do everything. Rather, look at it like a menu and add on something new every time you have your period, until you start to develop new habits and you see some of your symptoms shift.

Food	Exercise / Movement
• Iron: (heme) grass-fed beef, lamb, dark poultry meat, (non-heme) chickpeas/garbanzo beans, lentils, quinoa, kidney beans, kale	• Slow flow yoga, restorative yoga, yin yoga
• Vitamin C: citrus, kiwi, strawberries, raspberries, blueberries, broccoli, red pepper, yellow pepper	• Gentle swimming • Walking
	Lifestyle
• Copper: organic beef liver, oysters, potatoes, mushrooms, cashews, crab, sunflower seeds, dark / bittersweet chocolate	• Go a bit slower, if you can
• Magnesium: leafy green vegetables like kale, rocket/arugula, watercress and spinach; nuts, seeds	• Go to bed a bit earlier, take a longer bath and go into full self-care mode
• Vitamin A: organic beef liver, carrots, pumpkin, sweet potato, spinach, cod liver oil, spring/collard greens, kale	• Give yourself more time to get to where you need to go and to get things done
• Vitamin B12: organic red meat, dairy, eggs	• Give yourself space to ponder something that's been on your mind
• Omega-3: oily fish (SMASHHT), algae	
• Vitamin K: natto (fermented soybeans), chard, organic beef or chicken liver, spring/collard greens, spinach, kale, broccoli	• Use the box breathing exercise to help manage any pain or anxiety you might experience

CHAPTER 5

The Follicular Phase / Inner Spring

Every time I finish my period, I notice that there's a mental switch that gets activated. It flicks on and takes me out of my period cave and back into the hustle and bustle of my life. For many of us, once we've finished the hibernation of our periods (to whatever degree you allow yourself to slow down and rest!), there's a sense of being ready to jump back into our lives full pelt, with all the energy and a positive outlook on everything that's being thrown our way. In this chapter, I'll be taking you through the next phase of our menstrual cycle – the follicular phase, or our inner spring.

Mary's Story

Mary kept hearing her friends talk about how amazing they felt when their periods were over. She desperately wanted to relate and feel the same way, but she had always found this part of her menstrual cycle difficult. Her periods were really tough – heavy, painful and depleting. When they were over, she needed an extra week just to recover her energy and feel like herself again. And then there were the moods she had to deal with. As she moved closer and closer to ovulation,

Mary would feel a rise in anxious thoughts and self-doubt. She described this as the time when her inner critic came out to play. Then she would ovulate, and all would be right in her world again.

Mary went to see her doctor and was prescribed sertraline, an antidepressant, to help her get through this time in her menstrual cycle. She decided to try it for six months but didn't want to be on medication permanently. When the six months were over and she didn't feel much different, she got in touch with me.

Although her primary concerns were her mood and energy levels after her period, we needed to work backward and start by addressing her heavy and painful periods. The heaviness of her period in particular was depleting iron and copper, draining her energy and extending her post-period recovery time. We spent time addressing this (check out Chapters 4 and 8 to find out more about what to do if you have painful and / or heavy periods).

We then looked at how her body was responding to the rising hormones during this phase, in particular FSH, oestrogen and testosterone. We spent time supporting her liver and gut, using food and supplements to detoxify (or in other words, break down) the hormones Mary's body had already used. A part of this process was making sure that Mary was having regular bowel movements. She told me that she thought it was normal to poop every few days and that sometimes she could go up to four or five days without pooping.

As you'll find out later in the chapter, we want to poop every day. This helps our body get rid of the hormones it has broken down and avoids these hormones, especially oestrogen, being reabsorbed and recirculated back into the body. We increased the amount of fibre and fermented foods in Mary's meals to give her bowels a helping hand. These foods also helped her gut make enough serotonin and dopamine, the neurotransmitters that support our moods. We'll talk about the role of serotonin and other neurotransmitters later in this chapter.

I also encouraged her to drink at least 1.5l (3 pints) of water each day, as dehydration can contribute to constipation. We then added in lots of cruciferous vegetables such as broccoli sprouts, cauliflower, kohlrabi, asparagus and Brussels sprouts, as well as turmeric, ginger, citrus and high-quality protein like free-range, organic red meat and wild seafood to support her liver in the process of detoxifying hormones.

Finally, we looked at her lifestyle: how she was managing her energy during her whole menstrual cycle, how she was sleeping and how she was exercising. I encouraged her to look at energy a bit like a bank account – she needed to keep a positive balance. Constant withdrawals without corresponding times of rest would continue the cycle of depletion. I encouraged her to journal, especially during the times when her inner critic came out to play, and to write down the self-critical thoughts and examine whether they were really true.

Six months later, Mary said she felt like a different person. Her periods were lighter, less painful, and she didn't feel as depleted. She said that for the first time, she understood how her friends felt so good when they finished their periods, because she felt that way too.

Delving into Our Follicular Phase / Inner Spring

This is my favourite part of my menstrual cycle. I love the positive shifts in my mood, and I have bags and bags of energy to do everything I want to do. I feel stronger, I'm more open to taking risks and I'm more creative. But this phase of our cycles isn't all sunshine and roses. For some of us, as we can see in Mary's story, there can be a rise in anxiety, self-doubt and persistent low energy.

Let's look at what's happening during this phase of our cycle, which starts the day after our periods end. The follicular phase is when our body is focused on getting us ready to fertilize the mature egg that will be released during the next phase of our cycle, ovulation. When everything is going right, we have more energy, our skin starts to look fresh, plump and glowy, we feel brighter and more creative. We also feel more inclined to take risks in all areas of our lives. This is the time to start something new, big or small. You'll see a rise in your libido (and stronger orgasms!). There's a lot going on during this time.

Our follicular phase is generally the most flexible part of our menstrual cycle. It can last anywhere from 6 to 11 days, depending on the length of your entire menstrual cycle (remember, this is from day 1 of your period to the day before your next period starts). The variability in the length of the follicular phase is typically the main contributor to changes in the length of each menstrual cycle.[1] All this means is that you may ovulate on a different day each cycle – and that's totally normal. As we'll learn in the next chapter, just as not all of us have 28-day menstrual cycles, not all of us ovulate exactly on day 14. This is why it's vital to tune into the signs your body is giving you, including changes in cervical fluid, which we'll get into later in this chapter.

Having said that, our follicular phase can get shorter as we get older and move toward perimenopause (which typically starts in our mid 40s but can start as early as our late 30s!). A shorter follicular phase means a shorter menstrual cycle, so this is something to keep in mind if you start to notice your cycle length decreasing.

Let's get into the details of what happens during the follicular phase.

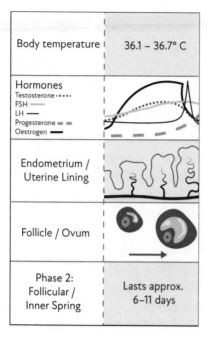

Body temperature	36.1 – 36.7° C
Hormones Testosterone ····· FSH ── LH ── Progesterone ▬ ▬ Oestrogen ▬	
Endometrium / Uterine Lining	
Follicle / Ovum	
Phase 2: Follicular / Inner Spring	Lasts approx. 6–11 days

What's Happening During the Follicular Phase

What's Happening Biologically?

This is the time in our menstrual cycle when our bodies are angling for us to do everything possible to maximize fertility. We're setting the scene to fertilize the mature egg during ovulation. Even if pregnancy is a long way off for you (or not on the cards at all), if you're cycling naturally without the use of hormonal contraception, this is the time in your cycle when your body wants you to look and feel your best in order to attract a partner.

If pregnancy is something that you're thinking about, now or in the future, you will be most fertile in the five days approaching ovulation and on the day of ovulation itself. "Why six days," you might be thinking, "if ovulation is only one day?" The six-day fertile window is due to sperm's ability to live inside the cervix for up to five days. Any sperm from the ejaculate gets pulled up into the uterus by cervical fluid. This is why I love it when my clients who are trying to conceive shift their focus away from the day of ovulation to simply having sex more regularly after they finish their period. It takes the pressure off (not many of us get turned on by overly scheduled sex, right?), and rising testosterone makes orgasms stronger, which pushes the sperm and cervical fluid further up the vaginal canal toward the uterus. And if you're going down an in vitro fertilization or intrauterine insemination (IVF / IUI) route, this is still relevant. Some of my clients have found it helpful when they understand where they are in their cycle, as it helps them connect the timings of the IVF / IUI cycle to what's happening to them personally. They're also able to ask more informed questions and feel more empowered through what can sometimes be a disempowering process.

During the follicular phase, the lining of our uterus (our endometrium) continues to grow, thickening so that if the mature egg is fertilized during ovulation, there is somewhere for it to implant.

What's Happening Physically?

I always notice the changes in my skin and hair during my follicular phase – it always seems like my hair is thicker and my skin is clearer and glowing. Do you notice this too? These changes are the effect of rising oestrogen.

You may also notice changes in your cervical fluid during this time in your menstrual cycle. Bear with me if this makes you feel a little squeamish. I would love it if we all became more comfortable with our bodily fluids, because we can get a lot of information from them about what's happening in our body. We produce cervical fluids at different levels throughout our menstrual cycle, but we start to notice them more toward the end of our periods, when we'll typically see clear, mucus-like fluid mixed with menstrual fluid.

As you move through the follicular phase toward ovulation, this cervical fluid starts to thicken and gradually turns the same consistency as egg whites. This is the result of rising oestrogen.[2]

Cervical fluid comprises fluid made by the cervix, water, bacteria (our vaginas have their own microbiome – a small universe of microorganisms, including bacteria) and cells from the wall of the vagina. This fluid has a number of different purposes, including:

- Helping to catch the sperm and pull them up from the cervix toward the uterus to give us a greater chance of fertilizing an egg that menstrual cycle
- Keeping the walls of the vagina lubricated
- Keeping the pH of the vagina balanced[3]
- Seeding the gut microbiome of the baby as it passes through the vaginal canal during vaginal births

If the cervical fluid catches the sperm before ovulation, it gets stored in cervical crypts, which are little glands in our cervix. These crypts are a cooler environment where sperm can hang out for a few days – this helps them survive longer! During our late follicular phase, the number of cervical crypts grows, which increases our ability to store more sperm.[4] Another reason why our bodies are so amazing!

Just a quick note: cervical fluid is different from arousal fluid, which (the clue's in the name!) is released when we're aroused. Because our libidos can increase as we move toward ovulation, we may notice that we might be wetter when we get aroused – that's the mix of cervical fluid and arousal fluid. We can produce arousal fluid throughout our entire menstrual cycle. It's produced by the Bartholin's glands (in the vagina) as lubrication to make sex, both penetrative and oral, easier.

Here are the changes you can expect to your cervical fluid through your menstrual cycle.

- Just after menstruation: some remaining blood / dry / sticky
- Early follicular phase: thick / sticky / watery / light yellow / cloudy / gluey
- Just before ovulation: slippery / creamy / egg-white consistency
- Ovulation: wet and slippery like an egg white, stretchy and elastic
- After ovulation: discharge decreases, can be thick, cloudy or gluey with more dry days

Basal body temperature (BBT) is another way to track your menstrual cycle and when you ovulate. BBT is typically taken just after waking to better understand the body's temperature after a period of rest. Before ovulation, your BBT averages between 36.1°C (96.9°F) and 36.7°C (98.06°F). If you are charting your BBT, you will ideally notice an increase to between 36.4°C (97.5°F) and 37°C (98.6°F), just after ovulation, where it will plateau until a few days before menstruation, when it returns to the lower range.[5] There are many factors that can affect BBT, including stress, an under or overactive thyroid, alcohol intake, sleep issues, pharmaceutical drugs, and even something as simple as the time you wake up or the climate you're in. If you want to learn more about BBT as a way of tracking your menstrual cycle, see a list of books on pages 297–302.

What's Happening Hormonally?
There's a lot going on hormonally during the follicular phase and what's exciting is how interconnected all these processes are. Let's have a look at how.

There are six major sex hormones that are active during the follicular phase:

- Gonadotropin-releasing hormone (GnRH)
- Follicle stimulating hormone (FSH)
- Oestrogen
- Luteinizing hormone (LH)
- Androstenedione
- Testosterone

All of these are driven by a set of processes called positive and negative feedback. Essentially, positive feedback is when our brain is told to produce more of a certain hormone. And negative feedback is the opposite: it slows the release of certain hormones. This feedback loop starts in the hypothalamus, a part of our brain that regulates the endocrine system (our hormone system) with the pituitary gland, another important part of our brain for hormone function.

Crucial to this feedback loop during the follicular phase is GnRH. This hormone is released from our hypothalamus in a pulse-like fashion and signals to our pituitary gland to release FSH and LH.[6] FSH is released in slow pulses, whereas LH is released in increasing pulse frequencies, leading to the LH surge at ovulation.[7]

FSH

FSH is the star hormone of this phase. It's been gradually rising since just before the end of your last period and starts to go into its peak just after your period ends.

The primary role of FSH is to recruit and stimulate a handful of Graafian ovarian follicles (otherwise known as mature ovarian follicles) in each ovary, one of which will become the dominant ovarian follicle, which then grows into a mature egg. This mature egg will be released during ovulation in the next menstrual cycle.[8] The selection process of the dominant follicle is led by a hormone called AMH (anti-Müllerian hormone), which typically declines as we get older.

Some of my clients who've been trying to conceive have been told by their doctors that a low AMH means that their eggs are bad or unhealthy. Setting aside the impact of hearing such disempowering words, it's critical to clarify the connection between AMH and fertility. Low AMH doesn't mean that all your eggs are stale, as one client was told(!). There is a lot you can do to improve the quality of your follicles and eggs, which we'll discuss in more detail in the next chapter. A low AMH result also doesn't mean that you won't be able to conceive naturally.

Additionally, FSH works to stimulate a set of cells in the dominant ovarian follicle called granulosa cells to activate an enzyme, aromatase. Aromatase then converts androgens (male hormones such as androstenedione and testosterone) into oestrogens (oestrone and oestradiol).[9] The dominant ovarian follicle starts increasing oestrogen levels, which then signals to the pituitary gland in the brain to slow FSH production.

Oestrogen

While FSH might be the star of the show, oestrogen is definitely one of the lead actors of this phase. As the dominant ovarian follicle grows, it continues to produce oestrogen, our feminizing hormone that helps the endometrial lining to grow. It also gives us that great glow and plumpness to our skin and makes our hair look bouncier. This is because oestrogen is linked with increased collagen production and more hydrated and thicker skin.[10] Oestrogen is also important for many of the structures in our skin to function well and helps wound healing. This means that you may notice a difference in the way cuts and wounds (and spots that you might have picked at!) heal in this phase of your cycle, compared to during your period, when your oestrogen is at its lowest point.

Rising oestrogen also has a positive effect on our immune system, giving us higher levels of antibodies (proteins in our blood that help us fight foreign invaders in our body, like bacteria and viruses) and a better immune response.[11]

As we learned on page 107, oestrogen is also responsible for increasing and changing cervical fluid and creating channels in the cervix that allow for sperm entry via the cervical fluid (the cervical crypts!). Oestrogen peaks about 24 hours before ovulation.

Oestrogen also works synergistically with testosterone to enhance sexual desire during the follicular phase.[12] Testosterone rises after menstruation, along with oestrogen. While our hormones *enhance* sexual desire, there are many other factors that affect our libidos, including energy levels, environment, sleep quality and mood. For many women, sexual desire is hormonal, physical and mental, which is why it's essential to understand the map of your own desire. What turns you on? What do you fantasize about? Do you know how to give yourself an orgasm (a fantastic way to reduce period pain, by the way)? Exploring the answers to these questions can help break down any mental barriers around desire and libido.

Luteinizing Hormone (LH)

As oestrogen peaks, our pituitary gland signals an increased pulse of LH, which stimulates another set of cells in the dominant ovarian follicle called theca cells. These cells produce progesterone and a male hormone called androstenedione. This rise in LH stops oestrogen production and starts the process of ovulation.

Androstenedione

Once androstenedione is released, it diffuses to the granulosa cells in the dominant ovarian follicle, which then bring FSH into action by converting androstenedione in the theca cells.[13] This male hormone doesn't have many effects, apart from its purpose in supporting the body's ability to convert it to testosterone and oestrogen.

Testosterone

Androstenedione is converted into testosterone in the theca cells in the dominant follicle, which is then converted into oestrone and oestradiol in the ovarian granulosa cells. It's amazing to think about how much is happening in these tiny cells!

Testosterone, one of our male hormones, is also important for women. As we learned earlier, it works with oestrogen to affect our sexual desire and libido during this phase of our cycle. You may also notice that you feel stronger or that you can lift more weight during the follicular phase. This is the effect of rising testosterone, which helps us maintain muscle mass, as well as bone strength.

What Are the Mental and Social Effects of the Follicular Phase?

When everything is working as it should, all the rising hormones during this phase will have a positive effect on our mental health. We'll feel more energetic, more confident and more creative. We're more open to newness in all aspects of our lives. Let's have a look at this in more detail.

Due to rising testosterone and oestrogen, as well as the brain neurotransmitter dopamine, you might find that you're more open to taking risks during this time in your menstrual cycle. Rising oestrogen affects the way that dopamine is released in the brain. This can potentially lead to an increase in risk-taking behaviour – which isn't always a bad thing! This is the time in your cycle where you may start to gravitate toward something new – a new job, a new project, even a new type of workout.

What does it mean to take more risks? It means that you're more likely to do something when you know there is a reward at the end of it. This reward comes with the risk of potential undesired consequences, but during this time in your menstrual cycle, the reward can outweigh the potential risks.

A 2019 meta-analysis of 23 published and 4 unpublished studies found that risk recognition and risk-taking behaviour is higher during this time in our menstrual cycle.[14] Some studies have found an increase in women's alcohol and tobacco consumption during the follicular phase, which is perhaps due to increased testosterone and dopamine levels. Interestingly, anecdotal evidence shows that this risk-taking behaviour declines after ovulation, due to the calming effect of progesterone and the brain neurotransmitter, GABA, which acts like a sedative, tamping down the exuberance of the follicular phase.

You may also notice that you feel more confident during this time of your cycle. This is the effect of testosterone, which also helps with an overall sense of wellbeing. If you're single and looking for a partner, this is the time to go on first dates. You'll be more confident and secure in yourself and that's always attractive!

If you have a pitch, presentation or talk coming up, try to schedule it during the latter part of this phase. Rising oestrogen is linked with rising levels of the neurotransmitters dopamine, serotonin, acetylcholine and noradrenaline. These neurotransmitters are associated with increased memory, communication skills and overall cognition. The research suggests that when we have sufficient levels of these neurotransmitters, the corresponding rise in oestrogen will also positively affect our communication skills during the follicular phase.[15]

Dara's Story

For the majority of her 20s and 30s, Dara's menstrual cycle was like clockwork. It was so consistent at 30 days that she was able to plan her wedding, honeymoon, house move and other major events around it. As she moved into her late 30s and early

40s, Dara started to notice that her cycle was becoming shorter and less regular. One month, it was 28 days, the next it was 26 days, then it was 25. For someone like Dara, who loved to plan and know what was coming next, this was disconcerting.

Dara came to see me on the recommendation of a friend who thought she might be perimenopausal. Although perimenopause can start in the late 30s, Dara was only 42, younger than the average age I would typically expect perimenopause to start. With this in mind, I wanted to work with Dara's doctor to dig into her symptoms more. We looked at blood, stool and hormone testing for more information.

I also wanted to understand how she was sleeping and what practices she put in place to manage her stress levels. Dara told me that she rarely went to bed before midnight and always tried to get up at 5.30am to get a jump on the day. She would brew a big pot of coffee and sip on this before eating breakfast with her kids at 7am. Dara said she would always get hangry around 10am and need to eat a snack so she could get through to lunchtime. Most of the time, she would be too busy to eat lunch, only eating once she started to feel lightheaded and a bit dizzy. Dara described her days as manic, juggling her business with school drop-offs and pick-ups, exercise, after-school activities and anything else that was required of her. After putting her kids to bed, she would buzz around, tidying up for the next day, before settling down on the couch with a glass of wine at 9pm.

I asked Dara to look at her schedule and see where she could ask others to support her. What chores could her children do to help out? How could her husband do more to take some things off her plate? Dara admitted that she found it hard to ask for help, often thinking, "I'll just do it myself." And her husband had long stopped asking Dara how he could help. Her kids were now seven and ten, the perfect age to be involved in household chores. I encouraged Dara to give each person in the household a daily chore and let them do it, without checking in on them. Dara also sat down with her husband to coordinate their schedules so that they could alternate school drop-off and pick-up each day.

I asked Dara to aim to be in bed and asleep by 11pm each night. We looked at her evening schedule and worked backward, looking at what she needed to change for this to happen. After a few weeks, Dara said she looked forward to her evening wind-down routine and was fierce about making sure this happened each night.

And, of course, we looked at what she was eating. Skipping meals and starting her day with a large mug of coffee meant that her blood sugar levels were on a rollercoaster, spiking her cortisol and putting her nervous system into sympathetic, fight or flight or freeze mode. All of this was a recipe for irregular menstrual cycles. Dara started getting up a little later at 6am and began to drink hot water and fresh lemon while she was making breakfast. I asked her to drink coffee with her breakfast and limit herself to two small cups. Breakfast shifted from a quick bowl of cereal to omelettes, porridge / oatmeal with nut butter and blueberries or green smoothies. I encouraged Dara to include enough protein and fat in her breakfasts to stabilize her blood sugar levels and keep her going until lunchtime.

We scheduled lunch in Dara's calendar each day as a non-negotiable. Dara started to put together quick salads with whatever she had in the refrigerator: greens, leftover protein from dinner or canned salmon or tuna, quinoa, grated carrot or beetroot/beet, some kimchi, salt and pepper and extra virgin olive oil and lemon juice drizzled over. I encouraged Dara to check in with her hunger and fullness signals throughout her meals so that she was able to stop overriding the cues her body was giving her to stop, eat and take a break.

After two months, Dara said that she was feeling much more energetic and less like she was running on pure adrenaline each day. And happily, her menstrual cycle started to regulate: the first month it was 28 days and then moved back to a consistent 30 days.

What's Normal During This Phase?

So far in the chapter, we've talked about the biological, physical, hormonal and mental changes that typically happen during the follicular phase. Again, when we talk about what's normal, this is what we would like to see if everything is working as it should. In this section, what I'll be describing as normal is what is biologically normal for this phase of the menstrual cycle. You may experience some of these changes, or you may experience all of them. Some cycles, you may experience the world at 100 per cent, other cycles you might be at 80 per cent due to other factors in your life, such as physical or emotional stress or lack of sleep. Remember, we're affected by what's happening in the world much more than we might realize. This will influence how we feel during each phase of our menstrual cycle. Here are some physical signs that are completely normal during this phase:

- Lots of energy
- A buoyant mood
- A relatively positive outlook on life
- Increasing libido
- A willingness to try new things
- Feeling more social or less introverted
- More cervical fluid that changes as we get closer to ovulation

- A smaller appetite, due to increased oestrogen
- Clearer skin
- Better sleep

As you move into the follicular phase and out of your period cave, you may notice that a cloud or a fog starts to lift, and you have a renewed sense of wellbeing. I personally love this phase of my cycle, but I must be mindful of my energy. I tend to overschedule myself because of this feeling of wanting to dive into everything. I like to think about my energy as a finite resource. If I use all of it now, I'll be depleted going into the week before my period and during my period, when I need it the most!

I will schedule meetings and presentations that require a lot of mental energy during this time, especially in the few days right before ovulation. Anything where I have to present my best self to the world, I try to schedule for late in my follicular phase. I am also mindful about what I plan a few weeks ahead of time. Far too often, my exuberance and zest for life during my follicular phase has meant I've made the mistake of taking my overscheduling into my late luteal phase. Inevitably, I end up with a diary I'm not happy about and a few days I need to rearrange. Have you ever done something similar?

What's Not Normal During This Phase?
There are a few things to watch out for that aren't normal.

- A short follicular phase (under six days)
- FSH levels still rise, but LH levels stay low, leading to more immature follicles that aren't ready to mature
- A long follicular phase (longer than 11 days)
- Imbalanced FSH and LH, which may be due to perimenopause or polycystic ovarian syndrome (PCOS)
- Your body may be making multiple attempts to ovulate, so your oestrogen and LH levels may stay elevated up

until a few days before menstruation; jet lag, lack of sleep and intensive exercise can impact this

- Anxiety
- Low energy
- Constipation
- Excess cervical fluid due to excess levels of oestrogen
- Very low libido

Take these symptoms as a sign that further investigation is needed. As we can see from the example of Mary's story at the beginning of this chapter, many of us can be taken aback when we experience problems in the follicular phase. We get told that this is the time when we're going to feel amazing, and it can be a bitter pill to swallow when we don't. What we eat, how we exercise and how we manage our stress can help us have a better follicular phase.

How To Improve Your Follicular Phase With Food

After we finish our periods, we start to reconnect with our bodies and there's perhaps a lightness as we move into our inner spring, a phase of renewal. I ask my clients to start to notice what foods they crave and gravitate toward during this time of their cycle.

As our hormones are rising, we want to do what we can to not only support these rising hormones, but also support the way our bodies eliminate them. Food is a fantastic way of doing this. This happens through a process in the liver and gut called hormone detoxification, where what we eat helps our liver break down our hormones to a less powerful form, to be eliminated through our bowel movements. Flip to Chapter 8 for a more detailed explanation.

This is why constipation is such a problem for hormone and menstrual health. Yes, there's some poop chat coming up! When we don't have a bowel movement at least once a day, it can impact oestrogen levels specifically and lead to excess oestrogen in the body.

You may be surprised, but the frequency that we poop is a bit controversial in the health space. Remember how I mentioned being really shocked when one of my nutrition lecturers said that we should ideally be pooping three times a day, after every meal? Conversely, some of my clients have shared that their doctors have told them that pooping once every few days is fine. Personally, I want my clients to have a bowel movement at least once a day, ideally first thing in the morning. Our livers and bowels are active overnight and a morning poop is a fantastic way of eliminating what our livers have broken down.

What our poop looks like matters too. In my practice, I use the Bristol stool chart (see overleaf), a diagnostic tool that breaks our stools into seven types, with the alternatives suggested by my nutrition colleague Clemmie Oliver. I'd like my clients eliminating stools that are between type 3 and 4, brown in colour and easy to pass, with no straining or excess wiping required. If you're a little stressed, your poops might be a type 2 or 5, but we're always looking for a baseline of type 3 or 4.

A quick note: certain foods can change the colour of your stool. If you've eaten a lot of greens, your poops may be green. Earthy red stools can be due to eating beetroot/ beet. If you have blood in your stool, please see your doctor.

You may notice that your stools change throughout your menstrual cycle. For example, you might get period poops, which are those softer, more frequent poops you might get before you menstruate. For some of us, they can be borderline diarrhoea. This is a sign of high levels of prostaglandins – read Chapter 8 for more information. You may also get constipated before or during your period. Try drinking more water, connecting with deep breathing to support your nervous system (stress can increase constipation!) and increasing the fibre in your diet.

The Bristol Stool Chart and Alternatives

Bristol stool chart			
Type 1		Separate hard lumps, like nuts (hard to pass)	Maltesers
Type 2		Sausage-shaped but lumpy	A bunch of grapes
Type 3		Like a sausage but with cracks on its surface	A Snickers bar
Type 4		Like a sausage or snake, smooth and soft	A sausage
Type 5		Soft blobs with clear-cut edges, (passed easily)	A broken 99 flake stick or Turtles
Type 6		Fluffy pieces with ragged edges, a mushy stool	Mushy porridge / oatmeal
Type 7		Watery, no solid pieces. Entirely liquid	Gravy

Let's have a look at the key nutrients and foods for a healthy follicular phase. As I mentioned in the last chapter, all the foods in each section have a particular benefit during this phase of the menstrual cycle, but they are also beneficial all cycle long. I've highlighted the benefits of the nutrients I discussed in the last chapter – and their benefits for the follicular phase – in the box opposite.

KEY NUTRIENTS AND FOODS FOR THE FOLLICULAR PHASE

Antioxidants: citrus, almonds, leafy greens, brightly coloured fruits and vegetables

Zinc: grass-fed red meat, oysters, mussels, clams, pumpkin seeds

Choline: eggs, fish, shellfish

Fibre: leafy greens, crucifers, nuts and seeds, fruit and vegetables with the peel on, carrots, sweet potato, quinoa, brown rice, brown pasta, brown bread

Phytoestrogens: flax, miso, fermented soy, chickpeas/garbanzo beans

Nutrient	Effect on Follicular Phase
Fats	The building block of progesterone, support the outer fatty layer of healthy eggs
Carbohydrates	Supports healthy energy levels
Copper and vitamin A	Helps us use the iron we get from food and supplement, supporting energy levels and blood rebuilding
Iron	Helps with post-period blood rebuilding and supports energy levels and mood
Omega-3	Can lower too-high FSH levels, which supports fertility[16]
Magnesium	Calms the nervous system, which is valuable for those that experience anxiety, helps the liver break down oestrogen once the body has used it

Antioxidants

You may have heard the term antioxidants with reference to skincare. They are also hugely beneficial for the health of our hormones and menstrual cycle. In a nutshell, antioxidants are nutrients that help fight damage from free radicals in our bodies. Think of free radicals as a pair without its partner – like Ant without Dec or Michael Jordan without Scottie Pippen. The antioxidant helps to make the free radical whole again, reducing the damage from the free radical. Antioxidants can help lower inflammation and support the immune system. This is important because our bodies want us to be as healthy as possible as we go into ovulation. While oestrogen is supportive for our immune health (remember that oestrogen is rising during this phase), too much of it can be inflammatory.

The good news is that you're probably already eating quite a few foods with antioxidants in them, like oranges and kiwis! These fruits are a great source of vitamin C, which is both a vitamin and an antioxidant.

An easy way to remember to eat more foods with antioxidants in them is to eat as many whole foods as possible. As you look through the list of antioxidants and example foods, I'm sure you'll start to notice a lot of crossover with other foods we've already talked about or will talk about in upcoming chapters. That's the beautiful thing about whole foods: they have so many overlapping benefits.

Antioxidants	Example Food
Vitamin C	Citrus, berries, broccoli, red and yellow peppers
Vitamin E	Almonds, sunflower seeds, avocado, spinach, kiwi
Vitamin A	Beef liver, sweet potatoes, carrots, cod liver oil
Selenium	Brazil nuts, shellfish, pork, beef, whole wheat
Zinc	Beef, shellfish, pumpkin seeds, lentils, chicken thigh and drumstick, oats
Copper	Shellfish, mushrooms, sweet potatoes, sesame seeds, hemp seeds

Selenium, a mineral that's also an antioxidant, has many benefits for supporting ovulation and good reproductive health. It helps healthy ovarian follicle growth and the growth of the ovarian granulosa cells (where we make oestrogen).[17]

Selenium is also critical to thyroid health because it can help lower thyroid antibodies, support thyroid hormone production and conversion, and reduce thyroid inflammation. We need about 55mcg (micrograms) of selenium each day,[18] which is easy to get from eating a couple of Brazil nuts.

When it comes to fruits and vegetables, a lovely rule of thumb is to eat the rainbow. Putting a wide variety of colours on your plate most meals will increase the number of specific types of antioxidants called polyphenols, which are plant chemicals found in most fruits and vegetables and are generally split into four categories: phenolic acids, flavonoids, stilbenes and lignans.[19]

Each colour has one or more antioxidants associated with it, so variety really helps. Here are some antioxidants you might find in some of your favourite fruits and vegetables and the associated colours. This is not an exhaustive list, so explore and eat the rainbow!

Antioxidants	Example Food	Associated Colour
Anthocyanins	Aubergine/eggplant, blackberries, blueberries, purple sprouting broccoli	Purple
Beta-carotene	Pumpkin, mangoes, carrots, apricots	Orange
Cryptoxanthins	Red pepper, pumpkin, mangoes	Red / Orange
Indoles	Broccoli, cabbage, kale	Green
Lycopene	Tomatoes, watermelon, pink grapefruit, strawberries	Red / Pink

Zinc

Remember how I mentioned the crossover in benefits from different foods? Zinc is a great example of this. We've just learned about zinc's benefit as an antioxidant. It's also an important building block for many hormones, including progesterone. Zinc helps the pituitary gland release FSH, which then supports ovulation and progesterone production. It also increases the body's ability to make progesterone.[20] Let's not forget testosterone: zinc also helps both men and women make this integral sex hormone.

Thinking back to our periods, zinc is a powerful anti-inflammatory, which means that it can help to reduce pain-based period symptoms. It also supports brain health, so it can be a great way to reduce cortisol and manage low moods.

It's fairly rare to have a severe zinc deficiency. However, dietary zinc deficiency is becoming more common, especially in vegetarians and vegans, because it's easier to get zinc from meat, dairy, eggs and seafood. It's also worth noting that some prescription drugs, such as the oral contraceptive pill and epilepsy medication, can reduce zinc absorption. The signs and symptoms of zinc deficiency[21] are:

- Low libido
- Loss of appetite
- Cuts and wounds healing slowly
- Getting sick regularly
- Thinning hair
- Low moods
- Slow recovery from colds
- Eczema
- Acne
- Anovulatory menstrual cycles, i.e. menstrual cycles with no ovulation
- White spots on fingernails

The recommended daily intake of zinc is 8mg, which is easy to get if you're eating a wide range of animal-based foods, because the bioavailability of zinc is higher in these foods. If you are vegetarian or vegan, I suggest adding in more foods that naturally have zinc, as it can be easier to absorb from food than from supplements.

Note that if you do take a zinc supplement, this can interfere with your body's ability to use copper. I typically recommend that my clients who need a zinc supplement only take it for three months maximum and do so at a separate time from food, in order to reduce the potential issues with copper absorption.

Iron supplementation can decrease zinc absorption, so if you are taking an iron supplement, take it on an empty stomach. If doing this makes you nauseous, take your iron with breakfast, when you are less likely to be eating foods high in zinc.

Example Sources of Zinc[22]	Milligrams
1 oyster	32.2
140g / 5oz steak	15
1 palm-size piece of beef	8.7
85g / 3oz cooked crab	4.7
2 tbsp cashews	2
2 tbsp pumpkin seeds	2

You can get zinc from plant-based foods such as nuts, seeds and whole grains, but a compound in these foods called phytate can reduce zinc absorption.[23] An easy way to reduce phytates is to soak or sprout your nuts and seeds before you eat them.

How To Soak and Sprout Your Nuts and Seeds

1. Cover your nuts or seeds in fresh, ideally filtered, water.
2. The harder the nut or seed is, the longer the soak time. Not sure? Soak for a minimum of 1–2 hours, or overnight.
3. After soaking, rinse, dry and store in an airtight container in a cupboard or in the refrigerator.

Choline

Choline is a lesser-known nutrient, but is key for supporting the health of your growing follicles and the maturation of the dominant follicle into a mature egg. It supports the quality of the outer layer (the cell membrane) of the egg, and the higher the quality of the mature egg, the more progesterone you'll produce. Choline becomes even more important in pregnancy, as it is needed to support the rapid fetal growth that happens over nine months.[24]

We need about 425mg of choline a day[25] and it's easy to obtain from free-range, organic meat, eggs and green vegetables such as broccoli and cauliflower.

Example Sources of Choline[26]	Milligrams
1 large egg (it's concentrated in the yolk!)	146.9
170g / 6oz steak	132.3
12 large prawns / shrimp	115.1
128g / 4½oz / 1¼ cups cooked Brussels sprouts	63.3
128g / 4½oz cooked broccoli	62.2
128g / 4½oz cooked cauliflower	48.8

Fibre

When you hear the word fibre, what comes to mind? Before I became a nutritionist, for me, fibre was bland, cardboard like foods or powders or pills. Basically, things that would help you poop if you were constipated! I now know that there's a whole world of fibre out there. The great news is that you're likely already eating a lot of high-fibre foods.

There are two types of fibre we need to know: soluble and insoluble,[27] which both come from plants. Soluble fibre can't be digested by the body and will dissolve in liquids. Think about how oats or beans go a bit mushy if they're left to soak too long. Insoluble fibre doesn't dissolve in liquids. We need both. They help make our stools softer and larger and keep us regular, which is important for our body's process of breaking down and eliminating the hormones it has used.

A cool added benefit of soluble fibre is that it acts like fuel for the bacteria in our gut, contributing to a healthy gut microbiome, which makes it easier to break down oestrogen in the estrobolome. The estrobolome is a group of bacteria and other microbes whose genes give them the ability to metabolize oestrogens.[28] In other words, we have special bacteria in our gut to help break oestrogen down. How amazing is that? The estrobolome also impacts the way oestrogen is broken down by regulating the way this hormone circulates around and out of the body through an enzyme called beta-glucuronidase. If you're constipated, you're likely to have higher levels of beta-glucuronidase, which will lead to oestrogens being reabsorbed.[29] You don't want this, as this can make period problems like heavy bleeds, mood changes and painful periods worse. In a nutshell: eat fibre because this helps you poop regularly, which helps your body get rid of the hormones it's used and broken down.

Sources of Soluble and Insoluble Fibre

Soluble Fibre	Insoluble Fibre
Oats	The peels of fruits and vegetables
Apples	Brown rice
Green bananas	Flaxseeds
Beans	Chia seeds
Psyllium husk	Whole wheat
Citrus	Nuts

We need about 30g of fibre a day, which works out to about five servings of vegetables and fruit. If we're eating the rainbow, this is an easy way to get a wide variety of high-fibre fruit and vegetables each day.

What's a Serving of Vegetables and Fruit?

Most of you will be familiar with the idea of eating five a day. In clinic, I love it when my clients eventually eat ten servings of vegetables and fruit each day – seven servings of vegetables and three servings of fruit. But what a serving actually looks like can be a real head-scratcher for some of us. Let me break it down for you! According to the British

Nutrition Foundation, a serving is 80g / 3oz, which is equivalent to:

- 1 medium apple
- 1 medium orange
- 7 strawberries
- ½ grapefruit
- 2–3 broccoli or cauliflower florets
- 4 heaped tablespoons of cooked spinach or kale
- 1 medium banana
- ½ medium avocado
- 2–3 asparagus spears
- 2 kiwis
- 1 large handful of grapes, cherries or berries
- ½ large white or sweet potato
- ½ medium cucumber

Phytoestrogens

Phytoestrogens are antioxidants that are a plant form of oestrogens. They are fantastic for helping to bring the oestrogen in our body back into balance (and supporting healthy cervical fluid). What's fascinating about phytoestrogens is that they work in multiple ways to support oestrogen balance, whether we have too much or too little. If you think back to Chapter 2, where we learned about the lock-and-key mechanism that governs hormones, phytoestrogens have similar chemical structures to oestradiol, the most prevalent form of oestrogen during our menstruating years. They can perform like weak forms of the hormone,[30] acting like another key to the lock of the oestrogen receptors on our brain, breasts, vagina, uterus, cervix, ovaries and more.

When you have too much oestrogen in relation to progesterone, phytoestrogens can stop those forms that are toxic in excess (known as 4-OH and 16-OH) from binding to our oestrogen receptors. When you are producing too little oestrogen in relation to progesterone, such as in the case of periods that are too short or too light, phytoestrogens can help bring oestrogen levels back into balance, by binding on to the oestrogen receptors that are missing a key.[31]

There are different types of phytoestrogens: lignans, stilbenes, flavones, isoflavones and coumestans. We can obtain these phytoestrogens from a wide variety of foods, including berries, cabbage, broccoli, seeds and legumes. When many of us think of phytoestrogens, we usually think of soy, which comes with a controversial reputation in the nutrition world, due to contradictory studies. Much of the soy that gets eaten in the Western world is unfermented and more processed, in contrast to the fermented soy (miso, natto, tempeh, tofu) that is mainly eaten in Asian countries like Japan. Think of the difference between soy milk and natto, which are fermented soybeans. Fermentation, similarly to soaking and sprouting, helps to reduce some of the anti-nutrients in soy, making it easier to digest and the nutrients in it easier to absorb.[32] When my clients ask me about soy, I ask them to eat a variety of fermented soy foods, alongside a range of other phytoestrogen foods, such as the ones below.

- Flaxseeds
- Carrots
- Broccoli
- Chickpeas/garbanzo beans
- Lentils
- Berries
- Fermented soy such as tofu, miso and tempeh
- Cabbage
- Dried fruits such as apricots, dates, raisins and prunes / dried plums

A Few Recipes for the Follicular Phase

I really love empowering my clients to feel confident enough to put together nourishing meals without feeling like they'll be lost in the kitchen without a recipe. This is where these simple meal formulas on the next page come in. You get a template that you can adjust based on your palate and favourite flavours. Don't like an ingredient I've suggested? Add an ingredient that you prefer instead!

Improving Your Follicular Phase With Stress Management

For everything to work as it should during the follicular phase, we need to have stress-management practices in place. I want to be clear about this – it's not just a weekly yoga class or a trip to the park. What I mean are the everyday practices that help manage cortisol levels and help our brain understand that it's safe for our body to produce GnRH, FSH and LH – that it's safe for our body to continue on its path to ovulation.

If we think back to Dara's story (see page 114), she was much more stressed than she realized. This was having a negative effect on her menstrual cycle, shortening her follicular phase and reducing the length of her whole cycle. Stress can be insidious and damaging, and to counteract this, our bodies are constantly working to bring us back to homeostasis, the status quo of our body. This is why we can be much more stressed than we realize. A great example of this is getting sick as soon as you go on holiday or even after taking a few days off work. Cortisol, our primary stress hormone, can suppress our immune system and tell our bodies that reproduction isn't important right now. This isn't what we want, especially during this phase of our menstrual cycle.

I believe that the things that we do, little and often, have the most powerful effect on our stress levels. Here are a few

BUDDHA BOWL FORMULAS

Grain (1 small scoop)	Greens and Vegetables	Protein and Fat
Quinoa	Chopped spinach, grated carrot and courgette/zucchini, roasted sweet potato and butternut squash, fresh broccoli florets, roasted broccoli, cauliflower, asparagus, plus 1 tbsp pumpkin seeds	Sliced grilled chicken seasoned with oregano, sea salt and pepper; or roughly grate 200g / 7oz tempeh using a box grater, then sauté in a pan until it starts to brown, about 5 minutes
Basmati rice	Kale and asparagus sautéed in extra virgin olive oil, roasted cauliflower seasoned with garam masala	Diced lamb sautéed in extra virgin olive oil, seasoned with sea salt and pepper; or 100–200g / 3½–7oz chickpeas/garbanzo beans sautéed in extra virgin olive oil or coconut oil, seasoned with sea salt and pepper
Couscous	Roasted broccoli, cauliflower, asparagus, grated beetroot/beet, topped with 1–2 tablespoons of hummus	Sliced chicken breast sautéed in extra virgin olive oil and minced garlic and seasoned with sea salt and pepper; or warm half a packet of pre-cooked Puy/French lentils and a pinch of salt in 2–3 tablespoons of water, draining the excess water once the lentils are warmed through

examples of small practices that you can incorporate into each day. Choose one and do it every day for a week and see how you feel.

- Start the day with a 5-minute reflective practice (resist the urge to look at your phone!). Think of one thing for which you're truly grateful
- Take a deep breath in through your nose and out through your nose before you start each meeting or meal
- If you have a desk-based job, stand up and stretch every hour. Don't be afraid to make it full-bodied, stretching your arms over your head and shaking your legs out
- Spend a few minutes savouring each meal. Really notice how it tastes – the flavours, the smell – and how it feels as you chew each bite

GOLDEN THREAD BREATH

Golden thread breath is a simple yogic breathing exercise that helps to manage the rising energy (and for some of us, the anxiety) that's associated with this phase.

Start by breathing in through your nose and exhaling through your slightly open lips. Do this for two breaths. Then, start to visualize a golden thread coming in through your nose as you inhale. And as you exhale, this golden thread will blow from your parted lips. The golden thread will get longer and longer as you lengthen your exhalation. Keep this golden thread in your mind's eye throughout this practice.

As you go through this breathing exercise, keep your face soft, your shoulders low and notice the shift in your nervous system.

Do this exercise for at least one minute to start and see how you feel!

Improving Your Follicular Phase With Exercise and Movement

Do you notice that there are certain times in your menstrual cycle where you feel more motivated, not only to exercise and move your body, but to try new types of exercise? That's the effect of rising testosterone and oestrogen and the desire for newness. Oestrogen contributes to higher energy levels and testosterone means that we feel stronger and it's easier to put on muscle.

High-energy workouts with a strength-based element are great to schedule in during the follicular phase. This could mean resistance training or taking a HIIT (high-intensity interval training) class with a weight focus. Or you could take a strong *ashtanga* or *vinyasa* flow yoga class that incorporates long holds or many *vinyasas* (love those *chaturangas* during this phase!).

If you're more inclined to focus on strength building, this is the time in your cycle when you'll not only be able to lift heavier, but you'll also notice that you might achieve more personal records. Go for gold!

With all exercise, it's imperative to both listen to your body and move in a way that feels right for you that day. Don't overdo it. Sustained intense exercise can have a negative effect on ovulation and can lead to longer menstrual cycles and in some cases, hypothalamic amenorrhea (missing periods), which we discuss in more detail in Chapter 10.

A Few Yoga Poses for the Follicular Phase

You may feel stronger and more inclined toward a strength-focused practice during your follicular phase. This doesn't necessarily mean you have to do handstands and forearm planks, although they may be easier to get into during this time. Here are some other poses with longer holds (at least ten counts) that will also help develop strength. Do each pose on the right and left side.

Tree / *Vrkasana*

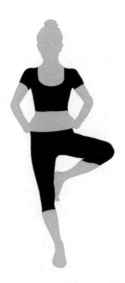

This pose combines strength, balance and focus, asking you to both lift from the crown of the head, whilst grounding down through your standing foot. To increase your focus, open up your arms to the side and sway from right to left, visualizing the gentle movements of a tree in your mind's eye.

Warrior 2 / *Virabhadrasana II*

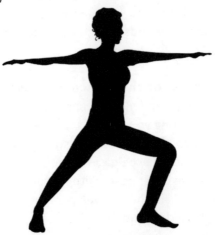

Warrior 2 pose asks us to tap into our inner and outer strength to hold the bend in our front knee and ground down into the edge of our back foot. Our outstretched arms increase the strength focus of this pose. Open your chest and roll your shoulders back, imagining you're holding a pencil in between your shoulder blades.

Triangle pose / *Trikonasana*

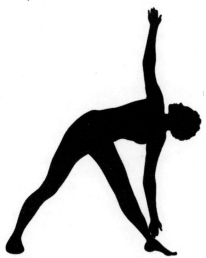

This is another standing pose that uses the core and legs to keep us upright and lifted. Imagine yourself balancing on a tightrope, your top arm pointing to 12 o'clock and your bottom arm pointing to 6 o'clock. You can add an additional core focus by moving your arms over your head pointing to 2 o'clock, imagining yourself holding a beach ball.

What You Can Try During the Follicullar Phase

Here's a summary of the different recommendations in this chapter. Don't feel you have to do everything. Rather, look at it like a menu and add on something new every time you move into this phase until you start to develop new habits and you see the changes you're looking for.

Food	Exercise / Movement
• Antioxidants: citrus, almonds, leafy greens, brightly coloured fruits and vegetables	• HIIT with a strength element
	• Strong yoga, such as *ashtanga* or *vinyasa* flow
• Selenium: Brazil nuts, shellfish, pork, beef, whole wheat	• Resistance training
• Zinc: grass-fed red meat, oysters, mussels, clams, pumpkin seeds	• Pilates
• Choline: eggs, free-range, organic meat and vegetables such as broccoli and cauliflower	**Lifestyle**
• Fibre: leafy greens, crucifers, nuts and seeds, fruit and veggies with the peel on, carrots, sweet potato, quinoa, brown rice, brown pasta, brown bread	• Harness your energy so that you are using the energy of this phase wisely
	• Try something new!
	• Use the golden thread breathing exercise to help harness energy
• Phytoestrogens: flax, miso, fermented tofu, natto, tempeh, berries	• Find a focus for the increased sexual energy!

CHAPTER 6
The Ovulatory Phase / Inner Summer

Ovulation is a reminder of how amazing our body really is. Every month (or however many days your cycle is) one of our ovaries releases a mature egg, which is the largest cell in the body, at a size of 18 to 25mm. From this one cell, we make oestrogen and progesterone (and increase the potential of having a child). I consider this phase of our menstrual cycles even more important than menstruation. If we don't ovulate, we don't make hormones!

I would love it if we shifted our focus from our periods. Instead, what if we focused on supporting healthy ovulation, so we're able to release as much progesterone as possible each menstrual cycle. In saying this, I'm not discounting the pain that so many of us go through during our periods. What we'll learn in this chapter is that by improving the process of ovulation, we can have a better menstrual cycle.

We'll look at what ovulation is, the effect it has on our body and what to do to make sure that you're ovulating well each menstrual cycle. We'll also learn that just as many of us don't have textbook 28-day menstrual cycles, many of us don't ovulate exactly on day 14 – and that's completely normal.

Finally, we'll learn about what happens when ovulation goes wrong and the unintended negative side effects of ovulation for some people.

Jennifer's Story

When Jennifer first came to see me in clinic, she believed she hadn't ovulated for a while. Her menstrual cycles were very long and irregular, averaging between 90 and 100 days. When she eventually got her period, she would have already experienced at least ten days of premenstrual symptoms, including mood swings, headaches, lots of crying, bloating and three or four days of spotting. Jennifer told me it was always such a huge relief when she finally got her period, even though she was also trying to get pregnant.

I had a hunch that Jennifer was potentially dealing with some form of polycystic ovarian syndrome (PCOS), and the hormonal dysregulation that underpins this condition meant that she wasn't ovulating every menstrual cycle. When we went through her health history, Jennifer displayed some of the classic signs of PCOS: she would feel hangry before most of her meals and if she didn't have a snack at 3 or 4pm, she would feel dizzy. She had even fainted a few times. Jennifer said that she could deal with these symptoms, but the dark, coarse hair (hirsutism) and cystic acne on her cheeks, chin and chest were a constant source of embarrassment. She couldn't believe she was still dealing with acne in her 30s!

I sent Jennifer to her doctor for blood testing so that we could understand what was happening with her oestrogen, progesterone, testosterone, sex hormone binding globulin (SHBG), FSH and LH levels. We also looked at blood markers related to blood sugar such as HbA1c and fasting insulin. I recommended that Jennifer have an ultrasound to assess whether there were cysts on her ovaries. The doctor agreed. It's important to note that the presence of cysts doesn't automatically mean a PCOS diagnosis. You can have polycystic ovaries without PCOS and you can have PCOS without ovarian cysts. As we'll discover in Chapter 10, PCOS is a collection of different symptoms that can be broadly classified into four types. Jennifer's blood tests came back showing that she was insulin-resistant, and her testosterone and cholesterol levels were outside the optimal range. There were no ovarian cysts on her ultrasound results. Jennifer's doctor agreed with my hypothesis of insulin-resistant PCOS and gave her the formal diagnosis she had been looking for.

We started by looking at ways to manage Jennifer's blood sugar levels to reduce the insulin resistance that was preventing her from ovulating. Insulin resistance means that the cells in the muscles, fat and liver don't respond well to receiving insulin, and these cells are unable to use glucose from the blood for energy. Jennifer's high insulin levels were connected to high testosterone, which was contributing to the hirsutism and cystic acne.

I suspected that high cortisol levels, which were the result of Jennifer's unbalanced work and lifestyle habits, were also exacerbating the insulin resistance and high androgen levels. Jennifer was one of those people who had to respond to an email or text straight away, even in the evening and at the weekend, often staying up past midnight with a tired and wired feeling and waking up early to jump on her Peloton bike. These habits led her to feel chronically stressed, with high cortisol levels throughout the day.

To get on top of this, we focused our work together on four areas: sleep, food, movement and stress management practices. I asked Jennifer to make sure she was getting to bed before 11pm each night, giving herself ample opportunity to unwind and relax before bed. We added more high-quality protein and fats to each meal to increase her satiety after she ate. This would keep her fuller for longer and reduce the need to grab a sugary snack for a quick energy boost. For the first month, I asked Jennifer to eat a snack at 3pm to get ahead of the energy dip that caused her to feel dizzy. We also redesigned her snacks so that she was eating combinations of protein and carbohydrates or fat and carbohydrates that would help balance her blood sugar levels. She began to add in snacks like sliced apple and cashew butter, chopped carrots and hummus and rice cakes and baba ghanoush.

Jennifer admitted that she was addicted to her Peloton, often taking at least six 45-minute classes each week. I asked Jennifer to begin adding in more variety to her workouts, swapping three Peloton classes for a class focused on resistance training, like yoga, Pilates or weight lifting. Research shows that resistance training increases insulin sensitivity,[1] so adding exercise that incorporated bodyweight or weights would help Jennifer's body become more sensitive to insulin, thereby over time reducing the insulin resistance and improving her blood sugar balance. I also asked Jennifer to spend ten minutes after all of her workouts cooling down and focusing on her breath, rather than jumping into the shower straight away. This would help tone her nervous system so that she could more easily shift out of fight or flight / the sympathetic nervous system to the parasympathetic, which helps us rest, digest, tend and befriend. This shift would help Jennifer better manage her cortisol levels and reduce a factor that was contributing to the insulin resistance.

We progressed by doing stool testing to pinpoint what factors in her gut microbiome were contributing to the acne. We discovered that Jennifer had a number of parasites that needed to be cleared and that these parasites were linked to acne and skin inflammation. Alongside a parasite-clearing programme that was tailored toward removing the specific ones found on the stool test, we also added in foods like broccoli, kale, pumpkin seeds, Brussels sprouts, eggs and free-range, organic red meat. These support healthy conversion of testosterone away from the hormonal pathway that is linked with acne and hirsutism.

Jennifer started to pay more attention to her energy, mood, libido and cervical fluid during each phase of her cycle. Six months later, Jennifer's cycles had shortened from 90 days to 50 days and she knew that she had definitely ovulated a few of those cycles. She was happy with her progress and this helped her to stay consistent. When I spoke to Jennifer a year later, her menstrual cycles had gone down to 35 days on average. Through a combination of basal body temperature and cervical fluid tracking, Jennifer knew that she was ovulating every cycle and she was more hopeful about the possibility of getting pregnant.

Delving into Our Ovulatory Phase / Inner Summer

When all is going well, ovulation is likely to be the time when we feel like our best self. The peak in progesterone and the second, smaller peak of oestrogen, along with the continuation of good levels of serotonin, dopamine and other brain neurotransmitters, contribute to a sense of being able to handle anything life throws our way. We're completely on point, we look great, our communication and creative skills are at their peak and our libido is skyrocketing. We're raring to go!

Although ovulation itself only happens on one day, I like to think of this phase as lasting at least five days. This includes ovulation itself and the release of our calming hormone, progesterone, and the second, smaller peak of oestrogen that happens after ovulation. As we'll learn in this chapter, the oestrogen contributes to continued high energy levels, while progesterone tamps down the fizziness that you might have felt during the late follicular phase.

Lara Briden, the author of the *Period Repair Manual* (2015), says that "ovulation is the main event of the menstrual cycle". I would love it if we put a special focus on supporting ovulation. Many of us don't know when we're ovulating or what the signs of ovulation are. We learn not to question it – we're simply happy to ride this wave of feeling good. As you read this chapter, I hope the information you learn will start to shift your emphasis toward ovulation and what you can do to support this valuable bodily function.

To put it simply, without ovulating, we don't produce progesterone. Without enough progesterone, the second, small peak of oestrogen rules unopposed, and this can lead to many of the symptoms we associate with PMS: mood swings, bloating, painful breasts, anxiety, headaches and depression. If we're not ovulating and we are having a period each cycle, this can have a detrimental effect on physical and mental health.

Let's find out more about what happens during ovulation.

What's Happening Biologically?

Ovulation occurs when the mature egg (also known as the ovum) is released from one of the two ovaries. Fun fact: we very rarely ovulate from both ovaries during the same menstrual cycle. When this does happen without the use of ovarian stimulation drugs like Clomid, it's called hyperovulation. This occurs when there is more than one dominant follicle selected to eventually turn into mature eggs, which results in more than one egg being released during ovulation. Some interesting research shows that mothers of naturally occurring fraternal twins (which are the product of hyperovulation) have been shown to have

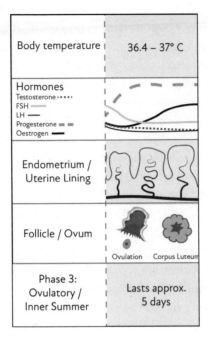

Body temperature	36.4 – 37° C
Hormones Testosterone ····· FSH —— LH —— Progesterone ▬ ▬ Oestrogen ▬	
Endometrium / Uterine Lining	
Follicle / Ovum	Ovulation Corpus Luteum
Phase 3: Ovulatory / Inner Summer	Lasts approx. 5 days

What's Happening During Ovulation

higher FSH or have a more frequent FSH pulse rate, thereby releasing more of this hormone during menstruation,[2] which can lead to the selection of more than one dominant follicle.

As we learned earlier in the book, the mature egg that's released during ovulation has taken about a year to grow to maturity, from primordial follicle to ovum. If fertility is something you're focused on, if possible, take a year to get your body and your follicles ready to start the process of trying to conceive. Usually, when we talk about supporting ovulation, we typically focus on the 70-day window it takes the mature (or Graafian) ovarian follicle to develop to be ready for ovulation.

When the mature egg is released from the ovary, it can be quite a violent process, which I know many find quite surprising. The egg has to break through the follicle and the wall of the ovary, an actual rupturing, because there are no holes in our ovaries. This is one of the reasons some of us may experience pain or spotting at ovulation. Ovulation pain, also known as *mittelschmerz* or middle pain, can feel different depending on the person, their levels of inflammation and even how the rest of the menstrual cycle is being managed. For some, ovulation can feel like a pinch or a dull ache. For others, it can feel like a red-hot burning poker on the ovary. Ovulation pain can also be a symptom of inflammation, pelvic scar tissue or another condition such as endometriosis, adenomyosis, fibroids or pelvic inflammatory disease. If you're concerned about chronic ovulation pain, please speak to your doctor.

Once the mature egg is released, it travels down in the respective fallopian tube toward the uterus, where it is ready to be fertilized by fresh sperm or the sperm that has been hanging out in the cervical crypts. If the egg isn't fertilized within 12 to 24 hours that cycle, it begins to degrade and becomes a part of what is shed with the uterine lining during the next period.

After the egg is released from the follicle, the remainder is called the corpus luteum, meaning "yellow body". This is where progesterone and oestrogen are released during the second half of our menstrual cycles. After it has finished its work, the corpus luteum gradually disintegrates and is absorbed back into the uterus. How's that for recycling? I will never *not* marvel at how efficient the body is.

A strong immune system is ticking along in the background supporting this process and ensuring the ovum is released into the healthiest possible environment. The rise in oestrogen during the follicular phase increases antibody levels and the strength of our immune response. This continues through ovulation with the anti-inflammatory effect of progesterone and the benefits of the second smaller peak of oestrogen.

What's Happening Physically?

If you're starting to become more aware of your menstrual cycle and when you ovulate, there are several physical signs of ovulation you can look for.

As we learned in the last chapter, our cervical fluid changes throughout our menstrual cycle. You may start to notice fluid that looks like clear egg whites. If you want to get to know your cervical fluid a little more, you can pick it up from your underwear or toilet paper and pull it apart with two fingers. It will be thick, stretchy and feel quite strong. This is exactly what we want – it's a sign of good health and is called peak cervical fluid.[3] This fluid is important for fertilization to take place, but it's also a sign that you have ovulated or are about to ovulate. I encourage you to get comfortable with your cervical fluid. Take your time, but eventually, I hope you are able to identify your changing cervical fluid and know when you're ovulating.

Another physical sign of ovulation is our basal body temperature (BBT), which we learned about in detail in Chapter 5. BBT increases just after ovulation, moving from an average of between 36.1°C (96.9°F) and 36.7°C (98°F) to between 36.4°C (97.5°F) and 37°C (98.6°F), where it will plateau until a few days before menstruation when it returns to the lower range.

The position of the cervix is another sign of ovulation. During menstruation and the follicular phase, the cervix will be positioned low in the vaginal canal and will be very firm. As we move toward ovulation, the cervix softens, moves higher in the vaginal canal and the cervical canal itself opens, in preparation for fertilization.[4] If you're not sure what position your cervix is in, you can check yourself or ask your partner. Toni Weschler, the author of *Taking Charge of Your Fertility*, recommends the following technique. Simply get into a comfortable squat, perhaps after your morning shower or bath. Insert your middle finger and use the acronym SHOW to check your cervix:[5]

S – Softness (firm / soft)
H – Height in the vagina (low / high)
O – Opening (closed / open)
W – Wetness (nothing / sticky / creamy / egg white)

Weschler says that it's best to start checking your cervical position after ovulation, so you know what a closed cervix feels like. Once you have this understanding, you can then start to check after menstruation to compare and contrast the position of your cervix at different times during your menstrual cycle. You may have no idea what you're doing when you start. Don't worry. It gets easier the more you practise.

What's Happening Hormonally?

During ovulation, our sex hormones are shifting, preparing us for either fertilization or to move into the luteal phase. There are three major sex hormones that are active during the ovulatory phase: luteinizing hormone (LH), progesterone and oestrogen. These hormones are responsible for ovulation and how we feel after we ovulate.

Luteinizing Hormone (LH)

The LH surge happens when the dominant follicle reaches a certain stage of development toward maturation. As LH surges, this can trigger ovulation, but not always, especially in perimenopause and PCOS. To know that you've ovulated, you should be aware of the physical signs of ovulation, which we talked about in the previous section.

Remember the feedback loop we learned about in the last chapter? Gonadotropin-releasing hormone (GnRH), which comes from the hypothalamus in our brain, signals the start of a positive feedback loop, which is needed for our pituitary gland to release LH. When we move toward ovulation, LH, starts increasing its pulse frequencies, begins surging about 12 to 24 hours after oestrogen peaks. The number of days that LH surges can vary: it can be a single peak, a double peak or a plateau that can range from 3 to 11 days.[6] This shows that just as the length of menstrual cycles can vary, so can the day that we ovulate. We don't all ovulate on day 14. This is essential if you get your serum progesterone levels tested: you want to test seven days after ovulation, not on day 21, because this assumes a 28-day cycle.

Progesterone

When we ovulate, we make progesterone, an important anti-inflammatory sex hormone that acts in opposition to oestrogen in the second half of our menstrual cycle. Think of oestrogen and progesterone like a see-saw. In the first half of our menstrual cycle, oestrogen is dominant. In the second half of our menstrual cycle, progesterone is dominant. Across our entire menstrual cycle, we produce much more progesterone than oestrogen, yet there is still a huge focus on oestrogen as the most important hormone for women. In her research paper "Women's reproductive system as balanced estradiol and progesterone actions: A revolutionary, paradigm-shifting concept in women's health", Dr Jerilynn Prior says that early research on oestrogen in the 1920s set the current cultural understanding of a dichotomy of oestrogen as the female hormone and testosterone as the male hormone.[7] Dr Prior argues (and I agree!) that progesterone is just as important as oestrogen. We must always focus on both hormones when we look at how we can support our health.

Later in this chapter, we'll discuss ways to support healthy progesterone levels and ovulation through food, supplements and lifestyle. Please bear in mind that everything we discussed in the last chapter about supporting healthy oestrogen levels will be applicable for keeping progesterone levels in balance.

After the LH surge that triggers ovulation begins, so does the pre-ovulatory rise in progesterone. This early rise in progesterone is important not only for ovulation itself, but also for the development of the corpus luteum, which is the ruptured follicle. Both LH and progesterone trigger the release of the mature egg, leaving behind the empty follicle, the corpus luteum.[8] This structure has a typical lifespan of 11–17 days, from ovulation to the start of our next period.[9] How incredible that our bodies can produce a temporary gland every menstrual cycle that makes such an important hormone!

Progesterone has a number of different functions:[10, 11]

- Has an anti-inflammatory effect in the body
- Regulates oestrogen levels by ensuring that oestrogen is not unopposed in the second half of our menstrual cycle
- Sustains pregnancy by maintaining the lining of the uterus and stopping contractions in the uterus that lead to the body rejecting the fertilized egg
- Supports GABA function in the brain (GABA is a brain neurotransmitter that has a calming effect)
- Has an inhibitory effect on sexual desire
- Supports a good night's sleep
- Has a protective effect on our breasts, reducing fibrocystic breast tissue
- Supports good mood
- Helps reduce bloating
- Plays a neuroprotective role in the central and peripheral nervous system
- Promotes bone growth
- Normalizes blood clotting
- Lowers blood pressure
- Regulates blood sugar metabolism by promoting insulin release after eating carbohydrate foods
- Helps us use fat and carbohydrates for energy
- Supports thyroid hormone function, increasing thyroid levels in the blood and helping more into the cells

Like oestrogen, progesterone is created from cholesterol in the ovaries, so we need dietary fats in our meals to help our body make these hormones.

Oestrogen

Oestrogen levels peak right before ovulation and begin to rise again after ovulation. This second, smaller peak of oestrogen rises in parallel to progesterone because it is also released from the corpus luteum.[12] This second peak contributes to continued high levels of energy just after ovulation, as well as the continued thickening of the endometrium in anticipation of implantation of the fertilized egg. To learn more about all the amazing things oestrogen does for us, flip back to page 110.

What Are the Mental and Social Effects of the Ovulatory Phase?

Ideally, this is the time in our menstrual cycle we'll feel our best. Oestrogen and testosterone have just peaked, our immune system is strong, our energy levels are still high, and we have the calming effects of progesterone to bring everything into balance.

The second, smaller peak of oestrogen means that we will still have significant, albeit lower, levels of the neurotransmitters serotonin, adrenaline, acetylcholine and dopamine, which will have a continued positive effect on our mood, motivation, memory, focus, attention and other cognitive skills. Progesterone also supports GABA production in the brain and has a calming, almost sedative-like effect.[13] This is where you may notice that the fizzing energy of the follicular phase starts to tamp down into something more calmed and controlled after ovulation.

This is the time to make the most of your heightened powers. If there is a negotiation element in your work, such as putting together contracts, selling something or even negotiating with a family member (convincing a child to eat their greens comes to mind here!), this is your time to shine. When my husband and I were buying a house, I joked that I wanted to time the negotiation to when I was ovulating so we could get the best possible price! Some studies show an improvement in verbal communication skills during ovulation,[14, 15] as well as a stronger memory, so you'll be able to pull out all the facts and figures you need for your negotiation more easily.

You may also find that you have increased emotional activity as you move through this phase, because of increased progesterone and its effect on the nervous system.[16] For those who experience premenstrual dysphoric disorder (PMDD), increased progesterone can have a negative effect, which we'll explore in more detail in Chapter 9.

I've mentioned the idea of thinking about your energy as a finite source. During ovulation, our energy peaks and it can be tempting to overschedule yourself. I encourage you to manage your energy during this time as much as you would during your period. Take breaks, connect with your inhale and exhale and use the progressive muscle scan at the end of this chapter to help reconnect you back into your body.

Cynthia's Story

When Cynthia first came to my clinic, she had recently become a vegetarian. She wanted to understand the best way to eat to have good energy and reduce heavy periods. As we dug deeper into her clinical history, Cynthia told me she suffered from terrible migraines that seemed to drift in about two weeks after her period started. Cynthia said that she could predict when they were coming because she would suddenly become hypersensitive to smells, she'd start sneezing a lot, her nose would get runny, and an aura would start to appear around lights. She knew that she would have to lie down, cancel the rest of her day and take her migraine medication, otherwise the headache would turn into a migraine and become a two- or three-day event.

I became curious about what I hypothesized were ovulatory migraines. I thought they could be connected to the pre-ovulatory increase in oestrogen and the corresponding increase in histamine levels. Histamine is a chemical that is made from immune cells called mast cells. At normal levels, they are a part of a healthy immune system, releasing as a response to potential allergens. Oestrogen stimulates mast cells to make histamine, which means that when oestrogen levels are too high, histamine levels increase as well.[17] High levels of oestrogen can also slow the way your body breaks down histamines, which can cause symptoms to persist.

Some of the symptoms of high histamine levels are migraines and headaches, bloating, nasal and sinus congestion, worsening allergies and itchy eyes and fatigue, all of which Cynthia experienced around ovulation. These would typically begin to abate a few days after ovulation, when progesterone levels rose and oestrogen levels reduced from their pre-ovulatory levels.

I wanted to address the migraines first, because these were having the biggest negative effect on her life. We started by putting strategies in place that would help to bring oestrogen levels back into balance in relation to progesterone. We increased the cruciferous vegetables in Cynthia's meals to support her liver in metabolizing oestrogen, we added more fibre so that she would have a daily bowel movement and we looked at the different skincare, make-up, personal care and cleaning products she was using and started to introduce natural and organic versions to reduce the amount of xenoestrogens (synthetic oestrogens) that Cynthia's liver needed to process.

I also gave Cynthia two supplements to help her manage the ovulatory migraines and the sinus-related symptoms: magnesium and quercetin. Magnesium is a relaxing mineral that can help reduce the intensity of the migraine and quercetin is a phytonutrient and antioxidant that helps to inhibit histamine release.[18] I asked Cynthia to up her consumption of high-quercetin foods such as onions, grapes, apples, kale, cherries and berries.

We also trialled reducing high-histamine food like red wine, kimchi, sauerkraut, dairy and chocolate (I know!) around ovulation to see if these would help reduce the intensity of migraines.

Over the next three menstrual cycles, Cynthia noticed that the ovulatory migraines were decreasing in intensity and felt more manageable. She said that she also noticed that her periods were becoming lighter and less messy. When I last spoke to Cynthia, her ovulatory migraines had decreased to slight headaches that she knew how to manage. This solution was a game changer that found her missing less work and finally enjoying the benefits of ovulation.

What's Normal During This Phase?

As we've gone through Jennifer and Cynthia's stories, we start to gain a better understanding of what isn't normal during ovulation. As I mentioned earlier in this chapter, I believe the ovulatory phase isn't just one day, but also includes the week or so afterwards when our progesterone and oestrogen levels are still high. If we incorporate the analogy of the seasons, this would be our inner summer. I love summer – to me, it really is the best season of the year. Everything feels bright, light and easy. As always, you may experience ovulation differently depending on what else is going on for you – your stress levels, your sleep, how you've been eating, how much exercise you've been doing and even how much you've been travelling. Jet lag can delay ovulation because it is a major stressor on the body. Our body needs to feel safe in order to ovulate, so anything it considers a stressor can influence ovulation and how much progesterone you produce.

Here are some physical signs that are completely normal during this phase:

- Lots of energy
- A calmer, more grounded mood
- More confidence
- A relatively positive outlook on life
- A slight increase in temperature
- Increased verbal communication skills
- Feeling social or a little less introverted
- More cervical fluid that is like egg whites in consistency
- Changes in appetite due to increased progesterone
- Clearer skin
- Increased appetite
- Better sleep

Remember: what's normal is a spectrum, but you should be able to sense a clear difference between how you feel during ovulation and how you feel during your period. Biologically, our body still wants us to fertilize the mature egg, so is doing everything possible to help us look and feel our best. Think about what you can do to take advantage of how you feel during this time.

What's Not Normal During This Phase?

There are a few things to watch out for that aren't normal.

- Ovulatory pain beyond the slight twinge or ache
- Headaches and migraines
- Exhaustion
- Brain fog
- Nasal or sinus congestion
- Excessive spotting

- No cervical fluid
- Constipation
- Not ovulating when you're naturally cycling
- Anxiety / depression / mood changes
- Bloating
- Increased allergies
- Worsening skin conditions such as eczema

When things aren't going right during ovulation or we're not ovulating at all, it can be frustrating. We're told that this is one of the best times in our menstrual cycle, our peak, and we don't feel like it is at all.

As we go through the rest of the chapter, we'll learn about what we can do to support ovulation and make sure that we're ovulating every cycle. As we get to the end of our menstruating years and toward perimenopause, we may find that there are cycles when we don't ovulate. This is normal. We have a finite number of follicles and as we get older, fewer and fewer follicles will go through the process of maturing into an ovum. If you are going through perimenopause now, the information in this chapter is still applicable, because you can continue to support your body through the cycles you do ovulate.

Improving Your Ovulatory Phase With Food

It can take up to a year for a follicle to go through the full journey of growing into the mature egg that is released during ovulation. What we eat will impact the health of the lifecycle of the egg: our follicles, the mature egg and the corpus luteum, which we know is important for releasing progesterone and oestrogen in the second half of our menstrual cycle. All of the recommendations in this book will help support this process.

We'll zoom in a little more in this section to focus on what you need to support the 70 to 90 days that the mature follicle takes to grow into the mature egg, or ovum that is released during ovulation. We'll also learn how to support healthy ovulation. When we look at progesterone, we need to consider its balance in relation to oestrogen. As we discussed, when oestrogen is too high or low in relation to progesterone, this has a negative effect on progesterone levels.

As ever, all of the foods in this section are beneficial during every phase of your menstrual cycle, especially if they are eaten as part of the Balanced Plate we went through on page 38.

KEY NUTRIENTS AND FOODS FOR THE OVULATORY PHASE

Vitamin E: sunflower seeds, almonds, avocados, kiwis, hazelnuts, spinach, chard

Vitamin B6: wild salmon, chicken, sweet potato, avocado, banana, jackfruit

Vitamin D: wild salmon, mushrooms, mackerel, canned salmon, milk, eggs

Probiotic food and drink: kimchi, sauerkraut, pickled vegetables, fermented soy such as tofu, miso and tempeh, full-fat Greek or plain yogurt, kefir, kombucha

It's worth noting that some of the nutrients we've talked about in the previous chapters have a positive effect on ovulation and progesterone.

Nutrient	Effect on Ovulation and Progesterone
Fats	The building block of progesterone, supports the outer fatty layer of healthy eggs
Carbohydrates	Support healthy energy levels during the ovulatory phase
Selenium	Supports the growth of healthy follicles and cells that release progesterone
Zinc	Helps us make more progesterone
Vitamin C	Helps support healthy follicle growth and increases progesterone levels
Magnesium	Helps decrease oestrogen levels, allowing progesterone to increase via ovulation
Vitamin B12	Low levels are linked with ovulation issues
Fibre	Helps us have daily bowel movements, which helps to bring oestrogen levels into balance

Vitamin E

When it comes to supporting progesterone, vitamin E is a powerhouse. It's a fat-soluble vitamin (along with vitamin A, D and K), which means we need to eat vitamin E foods with fats for them to work best. When we have too much of these fat-soluble vitamins, they get stored in our fat tissue. All other vitamins are water-soluble, so when we have enough, our body gets rid of the excess through our urine.

As we learned in the last chapter, vitamin E is also an antioxidant, so it's great to include during ovulation, when we want our immune system to be as strong as possible. In addition, vitamin E has oestrogenic, androgenic and progesterone-like properties, which means that it is beneficial for increasing and balancing these hormones. A small 2009 study found women with luteal phase defect or a short luteal phase (when the corpus luteum produces less progesterone than usual) who took 600mg of vitamin E three times a day from ovulation to the day before their next period increased blood flow to the corpus luteum, the structure that releases progesterone after ovulation.[19] Those studied also showed an increase in their serum progesterone levels (the amount of progesterone in their blood). Blood flow is hugely important for both the development and function of the corpus luteum, and without a healthy corpus luteum we won't produce enough progesterone each cycle. Be mindful that these are high levels of vitamin E, so if you feel your progesterone levels need to be supported, work with a practitioner to take the right amount of vitamin E for you.

We need about 8mg of vitamin E daily.[20] The best sources of vitamin E are from nuts, seeds and some vegetables. Smoothies that include leafy greens, avocado, nuts and seeds are a fantastic way to make sure you're getting enough vitamin E each day.

Example Sources of Vitamin E[21]	Milligrams
1 handful sunflower seeds	7.4
1 handful almonds	7.3
1 handful hazelnuts	4.3
180g / 6¼oz cooked spinach	3.7
156g / 5½oz cooked broccoli	2.3
½ medium avocado	2.1

Vitamin B6

If there was one vitamin I would recommend for bringing oestrogen and progesterone into balance, it would be vitamin B6. This little wonder is essential for our body to make the corpus luteum and it also supports detoxification in the liver by encouraging oestrogen to break down to its healthiest form, 2-OH, rather than 4-OH or 16-OH, which are stronger and in high levels have been associated with increased cancer risk. In doing this, B6 can help raise progesterone levels in relation to oestrogen. Vitamin B6 is also needed for our body to make the neurotransmitters that support our cognitive function, mood and sleep: GABA, serotonin, melatonin, noradrenaline, adrenaline and dopamine. It's also been shown to support the enzyme diamine oxidase (DAO) in reducing the high histamine levels that are behind ovulatory headaches,[22] which were part of Cynthia's story earlier in the chapter.

For painful periods, vitamin B6 can help reduce the number of prostaglandins our body is producing. A 2016 Indonesian study on 35 women found that 100mg of vitamin B6 supplementation for four days was able to significantly reduce period pain and prostaglandin levels.[23]

Vitamin B6 (along with the other B vitamins and vitamin C) is water-soluble, so we need to constantly replenish our body's supply through food and supplements. We need about 1.3mg of vitamin B6 each day, which you can get from food and supplements.[24] Eating oily fish a few times a week, along with sweet potatoes, squash and leafy greens are easy ways to get vitamin B6 into your meals. If you're taking a good multivitamin, with a B complex, you want to have at least 25mg of vitamin B6.

Example Sources of Vitamin B6[25]	Milligrams
1 medium cooked wild salmon fillet	1.6
1 medium chicken breast	1.6
245g / 9oz / 1 cup mashed sweet potatoes	0.6
1 medium avocado	0.5
1 medium banana	0.4
100g / 3½oz jackfruit	0.3

Vitamin D

As the sunshine vitamin (fun fact: it's actually a hormone!), vitamin D gets a lot of attention in the winter. Do you ever wonder why? 90 per cent of the vitamin D in our bodies comes from sun exposure and if you live in the Northern Hemisphere, you typically get the most vitamin D from the sun between April and October each year. Between November to March, the NHS recommends that we supplement to make sure we're getting enough vitamin D.

Vitamin D deficiency affects 50 per cent of the global population, especially those with darker skin, who need to absorb more ultraviolet B (UVB) in their skin than white people in order to make the same amount of vitamin D. This is due to melanin, the pigment in darker skin, which reduces the body's ability to make vitamin D when exposed to the sun. This means that those with darker skin require more sun exposure to produce the same amount of vitamin D.[26]

Why is vitamin D so important? It works alongside calcium, magnesium and vitamin K2 to help our bones stay strong and healthy. It is hugely important for hormone, menstrual, thyroid and immune health. D3, the active form of vitamin D, acts via vitamin D receptors (VDR) to regulate the expression of approximately 3,000 genes in various tissues, including reproductive tissues such as the ovaries, uterus and vagina.[27] When it comes to our menstrual health, vitamin D enhances ovulation by changing the signalling of AMH, the hormone that is responsible for selecting the dominant follicle.[28] It also increases FSH sensitivity,[29] which improves the health of our follicles and helps us make more progesterone.

If you experience period pain, check your vitamin D levels. Low vitamin D levels have been linked with painful periods[30] and can exacerbate chronic inflammation because of its powerful role in suppressing the prostaglandins that cause inflammation and period pain.[31] You might also notice that when your vitamin D levels are lower, you get sicker more often. This is due to the effect this hormone has on regulating our immune system.

Just 10 per cent of our vitamin D comes from food, in two forms: ergocalciferol (D2) and cholecalciferol (D3). Vitamin D3 comes from animal sources and is better absorbed and used by the body. This is also the type of vitamin D that is formed when our skin is exposed to sunlight. Vitamin D2 is mainly found in fortified foods, mushrooms (leave them on the windowsill in sunlight to activate the D2!) and supplements.

We need about 600IU / 15mcg (micrograms) per day.[32] During the warmer months, getting regular sun exposure will help keep your vitamin D levels strong. I typically recommend that my clients get about ten minutes of unprotected sun exposure each day. By all means, use SPF on your face, but keep your arms and legs (ideally your tummy and tops of your thighs as they are large panels that easily absorb vitamin D) unprotected. Let the vitamin D sink into the skin and then rub your sunscreen in. The app dminder is a great way to track your sun exposure and maximize your vitamin D intake based on the time of year and where you are in the world.

During the late autumn and winter months, I typically recommend that my clients top up their levels with food and a supplement of 2,000IU per day, taken through a spray on the inner cheek on the mouth or under the tongue that delivers vitamin D straight into the bloodstream. However, this is only after they get tested and we know that their levels are. Because vitamin D is fat-soluble, in other words, you store any excess amount in your fat tissue and you need to eat fat to absorb it; it's one of those Goldilocks vitamins we want to have the right amount of – not too much and not too little. I like to see vitamin D levels of at least 75 to 90nmol/l in my clients. You can ask your doctor to check your levels on a blood test or you can go to vitamindtest.org.uk and book a test directly.

If you get your levels checked and your levels are well below 75nmol/l, work with a practitioner to find the right supplement level for you.

Example Sources of Vitamin D[33]	Micrograms
1 medium cooked wild salmon fillet	28.4
100g / 3½oz / 1¾ cups sliced portobello mushrooms	28.4
1 medium mackerel fillet	18
1 can salmon with skin and bones	16.2
250ml / 9fl oz / 1 cup whole milk	3.2
1 large egg	1.1

Probiotic Food and Drink

When I teach clients about their gut health, I love using the analogy of a garden. We need seeds and fertilizer to help the garden grow and flourish. In the case of our gut, probiotic or fermented food and drink are the seeds because they introduce new strains of bacteria. Each strain has a different effect on our health: supporting our immune system, the breakdown of hormones in the estrobolome, our mental health and much more.

The fertilizers are the fibres we learned about in Chapter 5. Our gut bacteria feeds on this fibre, called prebiotics, and then produces short-chain fatty acids (SCFAs) such as butyrate, acetate and propionate. These help us metabolize carbohydrates and fats and have an anti-inflammatory effect, which supports our immune system.

Of course, it's helpful (and delicious!) to eat and drink these foods all cycle long, and during ovulation you'll have the additional benefit of giving your gut and immune system some extra love, releasing the ovum into the healthiest possible environment.

Some of you may already be eating fermented food and not realize it! Full-fat Greek or plain yogurt is an easy-to-access fermented food for many of us. Sourdough is becoming more popular, as are kefir and kombucha. And of course, these are traditional foods that are easy to make at home, like the ones listed below:

- Kimchi
- Sauerkraut
- Pickled vegetables
- Fermented soy such as tofu, miso and tempeh
- Full-fat Greek or plain yogurt
- Kefir
- Kombucha
- Buttermilk
- Sourdough bread

A Recipe for the Ovulatory Phase

Below I've included my recipe for pesto, carrot and sweet potato fritters. I love making these on a night where I want to cook but don't want to spend ages in the kitchen. If you use a food processor to grate the veggies, the fritters take 20 minutes tops!

PESTO CARROT AND SWEET POTATO FRITTERS

Prep and cook time: 20 minutes
Makes: 8–10 medium-size fritters

What you need:

5 tbsp extra virgin olive oil
½ medium onion, finely sliced
2 garlic cloves, minced
6–7 medium carrots, ends trimmed and grated
1 large sweet potato, peeled and grated
2 large eggs, beaten
3–4 sprigs fresh coriander / cilantro, chopped (you can
   use dried if fresh isn't available)
1–2 tsp sea salt
1 tsp freshly ground black pepper
50g / 1¾oz / 6 tbsp plain / all-purpose flour (you can
   also use gluten-free flour)
3–4 tbsp pesto, to serve

How to make it:

1. Heat a tablespoon of the olive oil in a frying pan or skillet over a medium heat and soften the onion and garlic for about 3–4 minutes, or until the onion is translucent. Remove from the pan and set aside, retaining the pan for later.
2. Put the grated carrot and sweet potato into a dish towel and squeeze out any excess moisture.
3. Put the vegetables into a bowl with the beaten eggs, sautéed onion and garlic, the coriander, salt and pepper and mix together until well combined.
4. Fold in the flour so it's fully incorporated into the mixture.
5. Heat the remaining olive oil in the pan over a medium heat.
6. Place 3–4 spoonfuls of the mixture into the pan and cook for 2 minutes on each side, then remove to drain on paper towels while you cook the remaining fritters.
7. Serve warm with the pesto on top. You can also make a garlic sauce for dipping: I like yogurt mixed with lemon juice and a little diced garlic.
8. Enjoy!

Improving Your Ovulatory Phase With Stress Management

In the previous chapter, we talked about the impact of stress on the follicular phase. This equally applies to ovulation. When the body is in a state of distress, our reproductive functions are downregulated because the body is focused on doing what it can to bring us back to our status quo.

But not all stress is bad. We hear so much about the negative effects of stress and how we need to reduce and manage it. Did you know there is a form of stress called eustress, or positive stress that can be beneficial? Eustress is often mistaken for anxiety, but it's those little bursts of adrenaline that can spur us into positive action. It's the excitement you might feel before going on a date, the thrill of organizing a surprise (and keeping it secret!) or the anticipation of starting a much-deserved new job.

We contrast this with distress, which we typically experience as chronic stress. It's working extra-long hours, not getting enough sleep, the heartbreak of a bereavement or a break-up. It's eating too much sugar, not eating enough or doing too much HIIT or cardio.

Eustress and Distress

Eustress	Distress
This is our body's natural chemical response to an exciting, new or stressful event.	This can make us feel overwhelmed
A temporary increase in adrenaline and cortisol	Chronic cortisol release which has negative effects on insulin, oestrogen and testosterone
Helps us stay motivated, excited and feel challenged	Can increase inflammation
Takes us out of our comfort zone	Triggers fight or flight response from the nervous system
	Negative impact on digestion, mood and sleep

As we learned in Chapter 3, our stress response system is governed by the HPA axis, and when we are overly distressed, it's the connection between these three organs that leads to chronic cortisol production, inhibiting gonadotropin-releasing hormone (GnRH), the hormone that tells our pituitary gland to release FSH and LH. This will have a negative effect on ovulation, leading to longer follicular phases, delayed ovulation and longer periods. Some research shows that high cortisol levels also negatively influence the ability of a mature egg to be fertilized.[34]

Be honest with yourself about the amount of stress you're experiencing right now. Can you distinguish between good stress and chronic distress? What are the small steps you're taking each day to counteract chronic distress? Our society puts 24/7 grind culture on a pedestal and many of us are now addicted to stress, always feeling like we need to be doing something, even when we're trying to relax. Think about how many times someone has asked you how you're doing, and you've responded with the words busy or stressed. It's okay not to be busy all the time. It's okay not to have a jam-packed schedule. Busy is not a badge of honour.

Try this progressive body scan to help connect you back into your body. Short on time? You can do an amended version of this scan with just your forehead and jaw. If you have more time, you can go beyond your face and add in the different parts of your arms and legs.

A PROGRESSIVE BODY SCAN TECHNIQUE FOR CONNECTING BACK TO THE BODY DURING OVULATION

Sit or lie down somewhere comfortable. If you are seated, bring both feet flat to the ground. Start by taking a long inhale and exhale in and out through your nose. Roll your shoulders back and relax your shoulders and hands.

1. Inhale and scrunch your forehead. Hold for 5 seconds. Exhale through your nose and release.
2. Inhale, squeeze your eyes and your cheeks tightly. Hold for 5 seconds. Exhale and release.
3. Inhale, clench your teeth and jaw, and stretch your mouth to a grin. Hold for 5 seconds. Exhale and release.
4. Inhale and make a kissy face by bringing your lips together. Hold for 5 seconds. Exhale and release.
5. Inhale and puff the air into your cheeks like a chipmunk. Hold for 5 seconds. Exhale and release.
6. Repeat a few times, if necessary.

Improving Your Ovulatory Phase With Exercise and Movement

Energy is at its peak during ovulation, so this is a great time to move your body in a way that helps you take advantage! The rise of progesterone and second smaller peak of oestrogen means that it's easier for your body to burn fat for energy. We metabolize more fat and protein during this time in our menstrual cycle, using more energy, which is why we might find that our appetite increases after we ovulate.

Oestrogen promotes glucose availability and uptake into type01 muscle fibres, which is the fuel of choice during short exercise sessions such as HIIT. However, progesterone can inhibit this, meaning that after ovulation, endurance exercise such as long runs, spin classes with endurance elements and swimming can feel easier and take longer to tire you out.[35] Adding in extra carbohydrate food such as sweet potatoes, brown rice and pasta, parsnips and pumpkin is a great way to make sure you have enough energy if you're planning to go for a long run, cycle or swim.

Please note that over-exercise can have a negative effect on ovulation and progesterone production. Generally speaking, exercise is supportive for many aspects of our health and wellbeing. The caveat is that when we over-exercise by doing too much (or too frequent) cardiovascular exercise, this puts additional stress on the body, increasing cortisol and telling the body that ovulation shouldn't be a priority. In my clients who are athletic, over-exercise and under-eating carbohydrates are the main reasons for lost periods. We discuss this in more detail in Chapter 10.

A Few Yoga Poses for the Ovulatory Phase

We're at the peak of our physical energy during the ovulatory phase. These yoga poses channel this energy, requiring us to focus on our inhale and exhale to keep us centred. Hold these poses for at least ten breaths or longer.

Goddess pose / *Utkata Konasana*

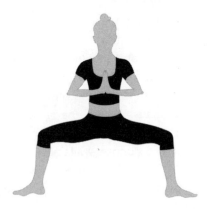

This is one of my favourite poses to practise and to teach. Goddess pose asks us to step into our power, opening the pelvis and hips, while bending our knees and grounding into all four corners of our feet. Once you feel steady, you can move your arms overhead, clasping your hands and releasing your index fingers. This is called *Kali mudra* and is known for helping us channel energy from our pelvis through the top of our heads and for cultivating strength and courage.

Wide-legged forward fold / *Prasarita*

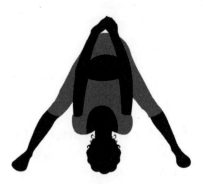

Prasarita pose is another strong pose that requires calm focus to hold. It helps us channel the strength and energy of the ovulatory phase. When I teach this pose, I offer several variations that enable students to challenge themselves, while also listening to their bodies. Starting with the feet wider than your hips, lift up from the pelvic floor and connect to the abdominal muscles to keep you stable, bring your hands to the hips and gaze down. You can add on by placing your hands on your shins or ankles, keeping your gaze in between your legs. If you want more, you can place your hands on your mat underneath your shoulders in line with the arches of your feet, keeping your weight in the balls of your feet. Gently come out of the pose by bringing your hands back on your hips and slowly lifting your torso upright.

Warrior 3 / *Virabhadrasana III*

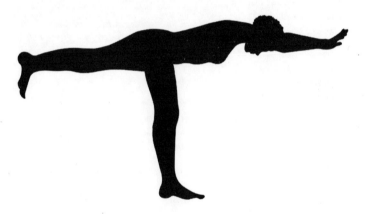

This pose combines balance and strength, asking us to ground into our standing foot and lift our raised leg as far backward as feels good. You might start by keeping the toe of the raised foot on the ground, gradually lifting to a place that's available to you. There are many options for the arms: prayer hands in front of the chest, airplane arms to the back or sides or outstretched in front. To increase your stability, focus your gaze on a point that isn't moving and hug everything into your centre. Hold the pose for ten breaths on the right and left side.

What You Can Try During the Ovulatory Phase

Here's a summary of the different recommendations in this chapter. Start by adding whatever resonates with you the most. Take a clear-eyed view about the different stressors in your life and what practices you have in place to reduce them.

Food	Exercise / Movement
• Vitamin E: sunflower seeds, almonds, avocados, kiwis, hazelnuts, spinach, chard	• Anything that helps you take advantage of the ovulatory peak of energy
• Vitamin B6: wild salmon, chicken, sweet potato, avocados, banana, jackfruit	• Endurance exercise such as long runs, cycles or swims
	Lifestyle
• Vitamin D: wild salmon, mushrooms, mackerel, canned salmon, milk, eggs	• Continue to harness your energy so that you are using the energy of this phase wisely – try not to overschedule yourself!
• Probiotic food and drink: kimchi, sauerkraut, pickled vegetables, fermented soy such as tofu, miso and tempeh, full-fat Greek or plain yogurt, kefir, kombucha	• Pitch for new business, schedule your performance review, have a conversation with your mentor, negotiate
	• Use the progressive muscle scan to help reduce cortisol levels and manage stress
	• Be social and connect with others

CHAPTER 7
The Luteal Phase / Inner Autumn or *WTF I'm PMSing!?*

Throughout this book, I've encouraged you to think differently about some aspects of your menstrual cycle. To look at your periods and entire menstrual cycle as one of your five vital signs, to get comfortable with menstrual blood and cervical fluid and to reframe ovulation as the true heart of our menstrual cycle. Now, I'd like you to start to think differently about the end of your menstrual cycle, the time most of us associate with premenstrual symptoms.

If you think about the cultural messages we receive from TV shows, movies, books and magazines about the week before our period, they're predominantly focused on women being bloated moody cows, unable to control our emotions or cravings. PMSing has become a loaded term that has resulted in many of us *expecting* to feel bad before our periods.

Here's the thing: just as I believe that period pain isn't inevitable, I feel the same way about PMS. It's not a done deal that we'll feel bloated, moody, depressed, anxious or (insert any of the many other premenstrual symptoms here) in the week or so before our periods. While it is true that some of us don't feel our best before our periods, we don't need to expect our mood and other parts of our health to fall to bits.

What we describe as PMS (premenstrual syndrome) is a collection of different symptoms that can affect us in the 5 to 11 days before our periods start. In this chapter, we'll learn what's happening physically, biologically and hormonally during this phase of our menstrual cycle. We'll talk about the mental and social effects, and we'll go through what to eat to help improve the luteal phase, especially if you're experiencing premenstrual symptoms. In Chapter 9, I talk about mood-based premenstrual symptoms in more detail, including anxiety, depression and premenstrual dysphoric disorder (PMDD), so flip to that chapter if those are specific concerns of yours.

Megumi's Story

Like clockwork, five days before Megumi's next period was due to start, her breasts would start to feel very heavy, with lumps and sore to the touch. Megumi would then rearrange her diary so she minimized any activities that caused her breasts to move a lot. Running and tennis were complete non-starters, and her boyfriend knew that sex was off the cards. Her breasts were simply too painful. She was fed up with feeling like this, month in, month out.

She had tried taking painkillers and doubling up her sports bra so that she could run and play tennis but wanted a long-term solution so that her life didn't stop for five days every month.

Because of the lumps in her breasts, I asked Megumi to see her doctor for an examination to rule out other possibilities, including breast cancer. We talked about regular breast self-examinations so that she could become more familiar with her breasts and how they felt during each phase of her menstrual cycle, and quickly spot any changes.

HOW TO EXAMINE YOUR BREASTS

The breast cancer charity CoppaFeel recommends checking your breasts regularly (at least once a month) and getting to know what normal feels like for you. You can check your breasts anywhere you feel comfortable, feeling them and anywhere there is breast tissue, including right up to your collarbone and under your armpits, in case there's any swelling. CoppaFeel suggest keeping an eye out for the following:

- If any areas feel thicker
- If any new lumps appear
- If there is a sudden change in size or shape
- If there is any dimpling or puckering
- If there are any unexplained rashes or redness

CoppaFeel also recommend checking your nipples, noticing if they've become pulled in, moved position, changed shape or if there is any crusting or liquid coming out (and you're not breastfeeding).

Very happily, by the time Megumi's appointment with the doctor came around, the breast lumps had disappeared. After an examination, the doctor concluded that Megumi had fibrocystic breasts (otherwise called non-cancerous breast lumps) and cyclical mastalgia, or painful and sore breasts. He recommended that she take painkillers to relieve the pain and that she continue to monitor her breasts, returning for further examination if the lumps returned or if there were any changes in the appearance of her breasts.

Although there are varying causes, the research shows that oestrogen levels that are out of balance with progesterone can contribute to fibrocystic breasts and breast tenderness.[1] I knew there were nutritional supports we could add into Megumi's meals to help realign her oestrogen and progesterone levels. Additionally, I wanted to address some of the nutrient deficiencies that were contributing to the premenstrual breast tenderness.

I asked her to do more to support her liver and gut – if you remember, this is where we break down the oestrogen our body has used before we eliminate it through our bowel movements. We looked at the different products Megumi was using on her skin, hair, body and to clean and scent her house. All of these would have an impact on her oestrogen levels.

Studies show that iodine can help with both breast pain and fibrocystic breasts,[2, 3] because it is both an important mineral for the health of our breast tissue and it has an anti-oestrogenic effect in the ovaries.[4] This is helpful when oestrogen levels are out of balance in relation to progesterone.

When working with clients, I prefer to start with food-based sources of iodine because iodine supplementation in large doses can have a negative impact on thyroid health. If you are considering iodine supplementation, please have your thyroid tested first to be sure you don't have an underlying thyroid condition. I asked Megumi to eat wild-caught oily fish (remember the acronym SMASHHT!) twice a week, add eggs to breakfast or lunch and snack on seaweed sheets at least three times a week.

As Megumi added in food to support her body's iodine levels and support the balance between oestrogen and progesterone, the breast tenderness gradually reduced over the next three menstrual cycles, and the lumps did not return. A fantastic result!

XENOESTROGENS

Throughout this book, we've extensively discussed how to balance the oestrogens your body makes in your ovaries, adrenal glands and fat tissues. Did you know that there is another type of oestrogen that can affect the balance between oestrogen and progesterone? Endocrine disrupting chemicals (EDCs) or xenoestrogens are manufactured compounds that, when absorbed by our body, get treated like the oestrogen we produce internally[5] and interfere with the way oestrogen normally works. These chemicals can bind to hormone receptors in the body (remember the lock-and-key process we talked about in Chapter 2?) and then activate, block or alter the way our hormones naturally work. There are over 87,000 chemicals in use today and at least 1,000 are recognized as potential endocrine disruptors.[6] EDCs have been associated with reduced fertility in men and women, period pain, disrupted ovulation, PCOS, endometriosis, thyroid dysfunction and more.[7]

Common xenoestrogens include:[8, 9]

- Bisphenol A (BPA): found in many plastic products
- Dioxins: a by-product of paper and cotton bleaching
- Perfluoroalkyl and polyfluoroalkyl substances (PFAS): used in non-stick pots, pans and textile coatings
- Parabens: found in shampoos, make-up, toothpaste, pharmaceuticals and food additives
- Phthalates: used to make plastics more flexible, found in food packaging and children's toys
- Triclosan: found in hand sanitizer and body wash
- Environmental pollution from airborne heavy metals and other pollutants

Whenever I talk about xenoestrogens, I always add the caveat that I'm not against man-made chemicals. Instead, I advocate an educated, empowered approach where you have a clear view about the influence of what you're putting on and in your body.

When I'm working with my clients, I ask them to do an audit of the following areas:

- Make-up
- Skincare
- Haircare
- Soap, deodorant and toothpaste
- Menstrual products
- Cleaning and laundry products
- Candles and room sprays
- Plastic food storage and cookware
- Cooking pots and pans

I then ask them to gradually start to incorporate eco-friendly, natural and organic versions of these products in a way that suits their budget. Don't feel as though you need to throw everything away at once. As you finish something, replace it with a hormone-friendly version. Check out the resources section on pages 297–302 for examples of eco-friendly, natural and organic products you might like to swap to.

Delving into Our Luteal Phase / Inner Autumn

I like to think of the last phase of our menstrual cycle as akin to autumn, when the days are crisp and bright and there's still a sense of possibility in the air. In our early inner autumn, our mood will still be balanced, and we'll still have enough energy to be able to do what we need to do. Then the weather begins to turn, the nights draw in and the leaves fall from the trees. In our late inner autumn, our oestrogen and progesterone levels are decreasing, affecting our energy levels and perhaps dampening our mood.

Our luteal phase can be one of the longest phases, lasting between 10 and 14 days. The timing of this phase can vary because we're sensitive to changes in progesterone levels: the more progesterone you produce after you ovulate, the longer this phase will be. Too little progesterone can bring our next period on sooner. When our oestrogen and progesterone levels are balanced (remember that see-saw analogy from the last chapter?) as we move to the end of this phase, we may feel like more muted versions of ourselves. That's okay! We're not meant to feel the same every day. When there is a hormone imbalance or nutrient deficiency, the dreaded PMS enters.

There are about 150 known premenstrual symptoms that cover the different systems and areas of the body, including our digestion, mood and emotions, skin, breasts, vagina and vulva, muscles and joints, bones, respiratory system, ear, nose, throat and the rest of our physical body. That's a lot, isn't it? When working with clients, I like to group premenstrual symptoms into five broad categories, ranging from mild to severe. Remember: these symptoms aren't inevitable and are indeed a sign from your body that something needs to be explored. If you experience some of the more severe premenstrual symptoms such as suicidal ideation, increased heartbeat / rate, shortness of breath and vomiting, please speak to your doctor as soon as possible. Premenstrual symptoms include:

- Pain: headaches, migraines, sensitivity to light / sound / smell / touch, muscle / joint pain, vaginal dryness, breast tenderness
- Mood: depression, anxiety (including increased heartbeat / rate and / or shortness of breath), anger, irritation, forgetfulness / brain fog, apathy, low motivation, avoidance, suicidal ideation (if you experience this, please

know that isn't normal and help is out there – please speak to your doctor or if you're in the UK phone the Samaritans on 116 123, and if you're in the US call 1 (800) 273-TALK), decreased resilience / ability to cope with day-to-day events, insomnia, fatigue
- Cravings: sweet, salty, savoury, chocolate
- Digestion: bloating, swelling, nausea, vomiting, increased / decreased appetite, thirst, sensitivity to alcohol and specific foods / flavours, water retention, dizziness, dry mouth, increased wind, constipation, diarrhoea
- Skin: acne, dryness, oiliness, increase in existing skin conditions, easy bruising

These symptoms can typically start between five and seven days before the start of the next period and usually abate when you get your period – or at least by day 2 or 3.

We'll cover premenstrual mood changes in more detail in Chapter 9, so flip ahead if you want help with these specific issues.

I want to reiterate that despite the huge range of premenstrual symptoms, we shouldn't expect to feel like crap just before our period. The late luteal phase can simply be a time when our energy decreases, we slow down a little, we feel flatter emotionally and that's it! We need to push back against the expectation that we'll be overrun by cravings, mood swings, pain, anger, bloating, etc right before our period, because similarly to period pain, we wouldn't accept this with any other condition, would we?

And before you roll your eyes and think that I'm being unrealistic, I'd like you to take a moment and ponder what it would feel like if your life wasn't being dictated by your premenstrual symptoms. What if you didn't have mood swings, rage or anxiety before your period? What if the only mood changes you experienced were normal human reactions to whatever's happening in your life?

Let's look at the luteal phase in more detail.

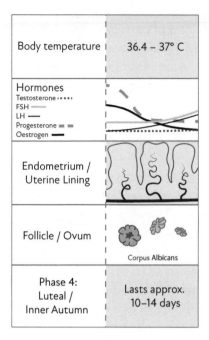

Body temperature	36.4 – 37° C
Hormones Testosterone ⋯⋯ FSH ⎯⎯ LH ⎯⎯ Progesterone ▬ ▬ Oestrogen ⎯⎯	
Endometrium / Uterine Lining	
Follicle / Ovum	Corpus Albicans
Phase 4: Luteal / Inner Autumn	Lasts approx. 10–14 days

What's Happening During the Luteal Phase

What's Happening Biologically?

If the mature egg that was released during ovulation hasn't been fertilized after about eight days, this signals that it's time to head toward the end of this menstrual cycle and try again in the next one.

The corpus luteum, the ruptured follicle from which progesterone and oestrogen are being released, starts to regress and degrade, with a total lifespan between 11 and 17 days.[10] It then turns into the corpus albicans, which gets absorbed into the lining of the endometrium. All the while, the endometrium (the lining of the uterus) is continuing to thicken in response to progesterone. The corpus albicans is shed along with the endometrium (the lining of the uterus) during the next period.

During the follicular and ovulatory phases, we learned about the protective effect of oestrogen on our immune system. The decline of oestrogen and the anti-inflammatory progesterone during the luteal phase reduces the strength of the immune system. Ever heard of period flu? This is why some of us may be prone to getting sick right before and during our periods.

What's Happening Physically?

When all is going well, we see fewer physical changes during the luteal phase. Our basal body temperature will have fallen, and we'll start to see less cervical fluid, especially in the late luteal phase when oestrogen levels are dropping.

There are two parts of the body where you may notice physical changes: your skin and your breasts.

Our breasts respond to cyclical changes in oestrogen and progesterone.[11] Oestrogen makes them look perter after menstruation by increasing the size of the ducts in the breast. They respond to the peak of progesterone after ovulation by increasing the stroma, the connective tissue in the breasts, which makes them look bigger. Progesterone also stimulates the formation of the milk glands in preparation for a potential pregnancy, even if you're not trying to get pregnant! During the luteal phase, when oestrogen and progesterone levels begin to fall, you might find that you lose some breast volume.

We can also see changes in our skin before our period, which, similarly to our breasts, responds to cyclical changes in oestrogen and progesterone. In Chapter 5, we learned about the skin benefits of the rise in oestrogen during the follicular phase. We may also notice a change in sebum or oil production during our cycle. In those who are prone to oily skin, the drop in oestrogen and progesterone during the luteal phase can trigger the glands that produce sebum, the sebaceous glands, to secrete more oil.

For those with skin-based conditions, such as atopic eczema, acne and hives, they can be exacerbated by this drop in hormones. This is because the skin barrier is more permeable just before menstruation, due to the loss of oestrogen's thickening effect.[12]

What's Happening Hormonally?

As the corpus luteum regresses and degrades, oestrogen and progesterone slowly return to the levels you would expect to see early in menstruation. This is why if you're using blood testing to check your hormones, you need to have them checked at the appropriate time in your cycle. This is especially important for progesterone. You may have been told to check progesterone on day 21 of your menstrual cycle, but this assumes that you ovulate on day 14, which we know is not true for most of us.[13] We want to test progesterone five to seven days after ovulation, when it will be at its peak.

When you're familiar with the signs of ovulation, you'll know when it's happened or about to happen. You can then book your blood test for five to seven days afterwards. Not sure when you're ovulating? You can use ovulation prediction kits (OPKs) to tell you when the LH surge is taking place. If you have PCOS, irregular periods or hypothalamic amenorrhea (when you haven't had a period for at least six months and you're not perimenopausal or menopausal), get your sex hormones checked at any time during your menstrual cycle.

When to Test Your Hormones

Hormone	When to Test
FSH, LH, oestradiol	Day 2 or 3 of your menstrual cycle (i.e. day 2 or 3 of your period)
Progesterone	5–7 days after ovulation
Testosterone, SHBG, androstenedione, DHEA	Any time during your cycle, preferably in the morning
TSH, T4, T3, RT3, TPO, TgAB	Any time during your cycle, preferably in the morning

Approximately two weeks after the formation of the corpus luteum, oestrogen and progesterone return to menstrual phase levels.[14] Remember: after ovulation, we're supposed to be progesterone dominant – progesterone is supposed to be high in relation to oestrogen. If there is an imbalance where oestrogen levels are higher than progesterone, this can lead to a number of the premenstrual symptoms listed earlier in this chapter.

Let's consider the impact of progesterone during the luteal phase.

In the previous chapter, we learned about the wide-ranging effects of this hormone (see page 147). When we don't have enough or any at all – and we're cycling naturally and not in perimenopause or menopause – this can lead to a condition called luteal phase defect or, as I prefer to think of it, luteal phase deficiency (LPD). LPD is a condition of insufficient progesterone exposure to maintain the lining of the uterus and allow for normal embryo implantation and growth.[15] This is the result of not ovulating that cycle or not producing enough progesterone during ovulation, which leads to a variety of symptoms, including a shorter luteal phase, premenstrual mood changes, spotting before menstruation and pregnancy loss. If you suspect you might have LPD, I recommend speaking to your doctor to check your progesterone levels.

In the meantime, go back to Chapter 6 and start adding in the foods that support healthy ovulation, corpus luteum formation and progesterone production. It's also helpful to look at lifestyle support, including getting better-quality sleep, addressing the factors that are increasing stress levels and moving your body in a wide variety of ways, especially those that support blood flow around the uterus. On page 201 I've included some yoga poses that are helpful for this.

As oestrogen levels gradually drop, so do serotonin and other neurotransmitters such as melatonin, dopamine, noradrenaline and adrenaline. This link is important because the drop in serotonin specifically can have a negative effect on our mood and increase anxiety levels, especially in those who already experience this.[16] Although the number varies, it's been reported that between 80 to 95 per cent of the serotonin in our body is made by the enterochromaffin cells in our gastrointestinal tract.[17, 18] To ensure that you're continuing to make enough serotonin so the premenstrual drop in oestrogen doesn't send your mood to the floor, keep your gut healthy with regular bowel movements, fibre, fermented food and breaks between meals to give your body time to digest. These breaks activate the migrating motor complex (MMC), the housekeeper of the digestive system, sweeping out anything left over from the stomach and intestines to be eliminated through bowel movements. Fun fact: the rumbling you hear in your tummy between meals is the MMC working! When in doubt, increase your fibre and fermented foods to support your gut. We'll talk about another great way to support your gut and serotonin levels later in this chapter.

We also need to consider the effects of cortisol, one of our stress hormones. As good ole progesterone and GABA, with their wonderful calming effects, start to decline, we would expect that the stress of the resulting changes to our mood, energy and sleep would increase cortisol levels. In the morning, we want cortisol levels to be high. This is what helps us get up feeling bright-eyed and bushy-tailed. If you're thinking, "That's never me!", cortisol will simply give you that impetus to get started with your day. Ideally, cortisol naturally declines as we go through the rest of our day, with our sleep hormone melatonin increasing in response to less daylight.

When it comes to cortisol levels during our menstrual cycle, an interesting meta-analysis found that the amount of cortisol circulating in the blood can actually be higher in the follicular phase compared to the luteal phase.[19] Of course, these levels will vary depending on individual circumstances and physical, emotional and systemic stressors.

What Are the Mental and Social Effects of the Luteal Phase?

In thinking about the wide range of women I've worked with, a common complaint is that the voice of their inner critic seems to get much louder during their luteal phase. Activities and tasks that they would normally feel confident about become subject to more second-guessing and doubt. For some, this can also manifest as being more critical about the way you look or even sound. Can you relate to this at all?

We talked about the inner critic in the follicular phase as the result of feeling overwhelmed by the rise in oestrogen, testosterone and neurotransmitters like serotonin and dopamine. In the luteal phase, this is the result of the decline in oestrogen, progesterone, serotonin and dopamine.

Ironically, I'm writing this section during my late luteal phase. I've really felt the self-doubt creep in and I've been having more and more critical thoughts about what I've written. When this happens, I find it helpful to stop, acknowledge these thoughts and ask myself if they're actually true – 99 per cent of the time they're not and 1 per cent of the time, the self-doubt and inner criticism force me to take a second look at what I'm doing and give it another sense check.

You might also find that you're less inclined to be social as you move further and further through the luteal phase, and you might be feeling a little less resilient.

It's not all bad news. Some of us might have a greater need to organize and nest during our luteal phase. We might get really focused on getting through our to-do list and "getting sh*t done" (GSD). In her 2015 book, *Moody Bitches,* psychiatrist Dr Julie Holland describes oestrogen as creating a veil of accommodation: we're more inclined to give to others.[20] When oestrogen drops right before our period, our tolerance levels decline and we're less likely to put up with anything we've been turning a blind eye to during the rest of our menstrual cycle. This also applies to the idea of GSD: Dr Holland says that during the late luteal phase when progesterone levels drop, we might be more dissatisfied with our current environment, and we may become more focused on making sure everything is set up for the next menstrual cycle. This includes any outstanding tasks. We just want to get stuff done. As I'm typing this, the image of the cartoon character Tasmanian Devil comes to mind.

If GSD at the end of your menstrual cycle resonates with you, you might notice that you have more energy to power you through your to-do list. Remember that energy is a finite resource. If you don't pace yourself, you may find that you feel even more tired on day 1 and 2 of your next period.

Akuada's Story

For as long she could remember, Akuada had to wear a larger set of trousers in the week before her period. Her normal trousers and jeans became too tight to button, and she would have to pull out what she called her "bloat trousers". This she could manage. It was the acne she found hard to take. Ten days before her period, large whiteheads would begin forming on her chest, cheeks and chin. Akuada said she found this so embarrassing and tried to cover them up as much as possible with thick foundation.

She wanted to have better skin, less bloating and have a better understanding of what was happening to her body every cycle. I asked Akuada to start keeping a food diary so I could understand what she was eating at each meal, what she was snacking on, how often she was having a bowel movement, the quantity and quality of her sleep and anything else that would help me understand what could be contributing to the bloating and acne.

I also asked Akuada to take a stool test so that we could have a look at her gut microbiome – the beneficial and not-so-beneficial bacteria, fungi, viruses and parasites that were hanging out in her small and large intestine. While we waited for the stool test results, I asked Akuada to pay more attention to the way she was eating. She had described rushing through most meals so that she could get on with her day. When we eat too quickly, we miss out on one of the first parts of digestion: chewing. Gulping our food down gives our stomach more work to do and we lose some of the benefits of salivary enzymes, which help break our food down before it goes further down our digestive tract to the oesophagus and the stomach.

I knew it wasn't going to be enough to simply ask Akuada to chew her food more. Before each meal, I asked Akuada to take a few deep breaths in and out of her nose, so that her nervous system would shift into the parasympathetic state, the rest and digest mode. This, along with the visual appeal and aroma of her food, would tell her brain that it was time to get ready to eat. Her stomach would start to increase its digestive juices in preparation for digestion. This would reduce the potential for bloating.

Akuada started to sit at the table to eat, rather than in front of her laptop, typing and chewing at the same time. The breathing exercise showed her the value of slowing down before a meal and she began to attempt to chew each bite of food at least ten times. Often, you may see other practitioners advocate chewing 30 times per bite, but I wanted this to be realistic for Akuada. She didn't have an hour to eat each meal and the thought of chewing her food to a paste each time didn't appeal. Finally, I asked her to put her fork and knife down between each bite.

After a week of incorporating these mindful eating practices, Akuada said she felt less bloated after eating and was a bit calmer too! When we received the stool test results, we found she had high levels of a bacterium associated with increased beta-glucuronidase, an intestinal compound linked to higher levels of oestrogen in relation to progesterone. When I looked through her food diaries, I saw that Akuada was only having one bowel movement a week, which gave her fewer opportunities to eliminate the excess oestrogen from her body. I suspected this may have contributed to Akuada's hormonal acne.

Constipation can also increase bloating because it prevents us from passing air and gas, one of the by-products of digestion. In addition, the drop in progesterone in the late luteal phase can increase the potential for bloating. I asked Akuada to increase the amount of fibre in each meal and drink at least 1.5l (3 pints) of water each day to help get things moving in the digestive tract. She started to have avocado with her morning toast, some edamame with her sushi at lunch and broccoli with her dinner.

After two months of making these changes consistently, Akuada was up to four bowel movements a week! She said that she felt less bloated before her period, her skin was clearer and by the time we finished working together, she had put her period bloat trousers in the back of her closet.

What's Normal During This Phase?

The American College of Obstetricians and Gynecologists estimates that around 85 per cent of women experience at least one premenstrual symptom every cycle.[21] When I talk to my clients about the end of the luteal phase, I always try to shift the expectation that we should assume that we're going to have premenstrual symptoms. They aren't inevitable. Oestrogen and progesterone levels are declining, so it is normal to have lower energy, a lower mood in comparison to ovulation and more hunger. What seems to throw a lot of us off is how hungry we get during our luteal phase.

There are three contributing factors to our increased hunger. During the early luteal phase, when our progesterone levels are still high, our body's ability to break down fat and protein increases,[22] which then can increase our appetite. There is conflicting evidence around whether we need more calories. As I explain later in this chapter, instead of focusing on calories, which are arbitrary and can burn differently depending on individual metabolism, I prefer for my clients to eat mindfully and increase the amount of protein and fat on their plates during their luteal phase.

The drop in oestrogen levels during the late luteal phase is connected with a number of different effects in our central nervous system, including changes in temperature regulation, hunger, mood and the way the body transmits pain signals. Interestingly, the neurotransmitter serotonin also regulates these functions.[23] Earlier in the chapter, we talked about the connection between serotonin and oestrogen. Serotonin levels rise along with oestrogen, pre- and post-ovulation. This is one of the reasons why we may feel pain differently at various points in our menstrual cycle. I always find that a toe stub hurts a little more right before my period. This is also another one of the contributors to increased hunger before our period. Higher levels of serotonin, along with oestrogen, have an appetite-suppressing effect after our periods end. This decline in oestrogen and serotonin starting in the mid-luteal phase stops the appetite-suppressing effect and contributes to increased hunger.[24]

We also have a significant decrease in GABA, the brain neurotransmitter that works with progesterone to calm our moods and produce melatonin, our sleep hormone. This is why some of us may experience premenstrual insomnia – we're already not producing enough progesterone and we don't have enough to help us ride the wave to the end of our menstrual cycle. This can manifest in poor sleep and mood changes.

Here are some signs that are completely normal during this phase:

- Increased hunger
- Declining energy
- Feel a little more self-critical
- Focused on what you know, rather than anything new
- Changing moods, potentially a little more flat or muted than usual
- Slightly more emotional
- Focused on completing tasks and getting through the to-do list
- Slightly tender breasts

What's Not Normal During This Phase?

There are a few things to watch out for that aren't normal.

- Excessive pain (flip to Chapter 8 for more support!)
- Constipation
- Diarrhoea
- Bloating
- Headaches
- Excessive breast pain and tenderness
- Swollen fingers, feet and face
- Anxiety
- Depression
- Angry outbursts
- Hot flashes
- Suicidal ideation (remember that you don't need to deal with this on your own. Please speak to your doctor or if you're in the UK phone the Samaritans on 116 123, and if you're in the US call 1 (800) 273-TALK)
- Vomiting

Improving Your Luteal Phase With Food

In our follicular phase, it's easier for our bodies to metabolize carbohydrates and we can be more insulin-sensitive, whereas during our luteal phase, it's easier for our bodies to break down fats and proteins. As we learned in the last section, this means that we can feel hungrier right before our period. As I always tell my clients: if you're hungry, eat!

Our protein needs are greater because progesterone decreases the levels of amino acids (what protein breaks down to) in our blood, and it also uses protein to help to thicken the lining of our uterus (the endometrium).[25] We use more protein during exercise, especially during the early part of the luteal phase when progesterone is peaking.

We also need to eat more fat during our luteal phase, especially at the beginning. This is because we need more fat to grow the lining of our uterus.[26] Dietary cholesterol is the backbone of oestrogen and progesterone, which we're making more of during the early luteal phase.

If we think back to the Balanced Plate on page 38, high-quality protein and fat are an essential part of each meal. If you make a habit of adding each of the four parts (fibre, greens, protein and fat) to your plate, you simply need to add a little extra protein and fat during your luteal phase. This will help address your body's needs during this time, support your blood sugar levels and help you manage some of the premenstrual cravings you might have.

Cravings are normal and are signals from our body that it needs something. It could be more sleep, less stress or a specific nutrient. I find it helpful to avoid treating cravings as something wrong or operating from a place of self-denial. I encourage you to do the same: examine the craving and give your body what it needs in a mindful way. If you crave chocolate, it can be a sign of the need for more magnesium, a mineral that can be depleted in the late luteal phase. And sometimes, you just want a bit of chocolate. Have the chocolate and enjoy it intentionally, noticing how it tastes and the sheer pleasure it brings to you.

Here are some typical premenstrual cravings and what they can mean.

Premenstrual Cravings and What They Mean

Cravings	Nutrient / Lifestyle Need
Chocolate	Need for more magnesium or tryptophan
Sweets / candy	A response to low blood sugar and / or high cortisol. Increase protein and fat to help balance blood sugar levels. Increase magnesium, chromium and potassium
Salt	Can be the result of chronic stress and / or excessive sweating. Replace sodium and potassium
Simple carbohydrates (white bread, rice, pasta)	Can temporarily increase serotonin, the neurotransmitter that is associated with happiness, which gradually declines during the luteal phase

KEY NUTRIENTS AND FOODS FOR THE LUTEAL PHASE

Tryptophan: poultry, red meat, pork, salmon, beans, pumpkin seeds, oats, eggs

Calcium: sardines, salmon, full-fat yogurt, whole milk, cheese, tahini, spinach, black-eyed beans / peas, almonds

Potassium: potatoes, apricots, prunes / dried plums, banana, artichokes, oranges, sunflower seeds, eggs

Iodine: seaweed, cod, potatoes (especially the ones from Jersey!), prawns / shrimp, whole milk, eggs, tuna, strawberries

It's also worth noting that some of the nutrients we've talked about in the previous chapters have a positive effect during the luteal phase.

Nutrient	Effect on Luteal Phase
Protein	Increased protein metabolism increases protein requirements during the luteal phase[27]
Fat	Increased fat metabolism increases fat requirements in the luteal phase
Vitamin C	Supports progesterone production, helpful for luteal phase deficiency[28]
Vitamin E	Supports progesterone production, helpful for breast pain, helpful for luteal phase deficiency[29]
Omega-3	Helps reduce inflammation
Magnesium	Supports energy levels and mood, helps to reduce premenstrual cramping, breast tenderness and headaches, reduces chocolate cravings
Vitamin B6	Supports serotonin and dopamine production, encourages healthy balance between oestrogen and progesterone, supports transfer of magnesium into cells
Iron	Important for tryptophan conversion into serotonin
Fibre and fermented foods	Supports oestrogen clearance and excretion
Vitamin B2 (riboflavin)	Required to convert B6 to a useable form in the body
Vitamin B3 (niacin)	Reduces tryptophan depletion
Vitamin B12	Required to metabolize serotonin and dopamine
Vitamin B9 (folate)	Required to metabolize serotonin and dopamine

Tryptophan

When it comes to making serotonin, it's not just gut health we need to focus on. Tryptophan, one of the nine essential amino acids that combine to form protein, is required for our bodies to make enough serotonin. We can't make tryptophan ourselves, so we need to get it from the food we eat.

Adding tryptophan foods into our meals during the luteal phase can help our bodies continue to make enough serotonin, which can then help improve our mood. To get the full benefit of tryptophan foods, it's best to eat them alongside complex carbohydrates such as sweet potatoes, brown rice, brown pasta, pumpkin, carrots and chickpeas/garbanzo beans. This also helps manage our blood sugar levels and avoid the energy crashes that can worsen our mood and contribute to anxiety.

Example Sources of Tryptophan[30]	Milligrams
1 hand-size chicken breast (170g / 6oz)	687
1 hand-size steak (170g / 6oz)	636
1 hand-size pork chop (170g / 6oz)	627
1 hand-size portion salmon (170g / 6oz)	570
1 hand-size portion roast turkey (170g / 6oz)	507
150g / 5½oz / 1 cup red kidney beans	198
1 handful pumpkin seeds	164
1 large egg	77
100g / 3½oz cooked porridge / oatmeal	40

Calcium

There's a strong link between calcium (and magnesium, and vitamins D and K!) and bone health. When I was growing up, there were commercials on TV telling us how important milk and calcium are for strong, healthy bones. Remember the Got Milk? campaign with all the celebrities sporting milk moustaches?

Keeping our bones strong throughout our menstruating years helps reduce the risk of osteoporosis, which increases after menopause,[31] because of the decrease in bone protective levels of oestrogen.[32] Eating enough calcium, magnesium, vitamin D and vitamin K foods will support bone health, as will regular weight-bearing exercise that helps the bone break down and rebuild again.

Looking beyond bone health, getting enough calcium in our meals is also valuable for reducing premenstrual symptoms. Research has found that low levels of calcium in our blood can cause or exacerbate premenstrual symptoms in the late luteal phase.[33] Interestingly, there is some evidence that calcium levels are significantly higher in the follicular phase because of the increase of oestrogen,[34] which is one of the reasons why, in my clinical nutrition practice, I move my clients toward increasing calcium levels through food rather than through supplements – because of the risk of kidney stones and digestive issues from overly high calcium levels.

We need about 1,000mg of calcium each day,[35] which we can get from a wide variety of food. And it's not just the dairy sources like milk, yogurt and cheese, as we may have learned in elementary school. Dark leafy greens, almonds, sesame seeds, sardines and other small fish are a great source of calcium – as long as you eat the bones!

Example Sources of Calcium[36]	Milligrams
A can of sardines (100g / 3½oz)	430
A can of salmon (120g / 4¼oz)	360
1 cup plain yogurt (240g / 8oz)	297
1 small glass whole cow's milk (230ml / 7¾fl oz)	293
Matchstick-size piece of Gruyère cheese (13g / ½oz)	287
2 tbsp tahini	260
100g / 3½oz raw kale	150
100g / 3½oz cooked spinach	136
100g / 3½oz / 150g / 5½oz black-eyed beans / peas	128
10 whole almonds (40g / 1½oz)	92

Potassium

If anyone asks me about underrated minerals, potassium features high on the list. When we don't have enough of it, it affects our hydration levels, energy and even how much we crave sweets! Potassium works hand in hand with sodium as electrolyte minerals that help our cells work their best and maintain fluid balance in the body. Potassium takes water out of cells and sodium pulls it into cells. When we don't have enough potassium in our meals, it can make us a little more sensitive to salt and changes in blood pressure.

When it comes to our menstrual health, adding more potassium-rich food is helpful for several reasons. It helps with the optimal production of progesterone after the LH surge and helps reduce hydration- and bloating-related premenstrual symptoms.

We need about 2,320mg of potassium each day.[37] Like zinc, sodium and magnesium, our potassium levels can fluctuate across the menstrual cycle.[38] Although potassium levels can be higher during our luteal phase,[39] you may not have enough to begin with, which can lead to premenstrual symptoms such as bloating and swollen fingers and feet. If you find that you get bloated before your period, try adding in some common potassium foods like baked potatoes, bananas and oranges!

Example Sources of Potassium[40]	Milligrams
1 medium baked potato with the skin	926
10 dried apricots	755
10 prunes / dried plums	637
1 medium banana	422
1 medium cooked artichoke	343
1 medium orange	238
3 tbsp sunflower seeds	137
1 large egg	81

Sodium

Let's talk about potassium's sister mineral, sodium. I think sodium has a bad reputation. We need to have some sodium in our meals, not only for flavour, but also to help our cells stay hydrated. The challenge is that many processed foods and restaurant meals have higher-than-necessary levels to help boost the flavour.

We want to find a middle ground with sodium – not too much and not too little. Too much can affect our blood pressure and the way our muscles and nerves function.

We need about 6g of sodium each day,[41] which we can get from many whole foods. Think about seaweed, fish and shellfish, with their naturally salty taste, or eggs, celery or artichokes. The natural sodium in these foods is different from the salt that we add in for flavour or to preserve.

As with potassium, high sodium levels can lead to premenstrual bloating and water retention. If this is an issue for you, take a look at two areas: how much extra salt you're adding to your food when you cook and how much high-sodium packaged and processed foods you're eating.

Iodine

In Megumi's story on page 172, we learned about the benefits of iodine for breast health, including how foods with iodine can help reduce premenstrual breast tenderness and pain because of its role in promoting the growth of normal breast tissue.[42] Iodine is also helpful if you have breast tenderness or pain around ovulation. It's always important to act cautiously when it comes to our breasts. If you notice any significant changes in your breasts, including size, texture, nipple shape, discharge or lumps, please speak to your doctor. The lumps may be a condition called fibrocystic breasts, when benign lumps appear around ovulation or before menstruation, but it's always valuable to rule out any other conditions, especially if you have a family history of breast cancer.

Iodine is also an important part of the way our thyroid, the butterfly-shaped gland at the base of our throat, functions. In many countries around the world, including the UK, mild iodine deficiency is an issue.[43] When it comes to menstrual health, the health of our thyroid is intricately connected. Underconsumption of iodine, which is necessary to form the thyroid hormones T4 and T3, can result in hypothyroidism, a condition where the thyroid gland is underactive. This can lead to fatigue, hair loss, cold hands and feet, dry skin, heavy and / or irregular periods.

We need about 150mcg (micrograms) of iodine a day,[44] which we can get from food and supplements. If you are a vegetarian or a vegan, it's crucial to be intentional about including sources of iodine in your meals. Seaweed, strawberries and Jersey potatoes are great options to include, but remember that because it has high iodine levels, a little seaweed can go a long way. Here's a fun fact: farmers in Jersey, Ireland and maritime Canada fertilize their fields with seaweed, which is why their potatoes are such a great source of iodine!

Example Sources of Iodine[45]	Micrograms
1 pack of small dried seaweed sheets (10g / 1 / 3oz)	232
A playing-card-size piece of cod	158
1 medium baked potato with the skin	60
9 prawns / shrimp	35
1 small glass of whole milk (230ml / 7¾fl oz)	28
1 large egg	25
½ can of tuna	17
6–7 strawberries	12

A Recipe for the Luteal Phase

I've included my recipe for peanut butter cookies on the next page. If you fancy a sweet treat before your period, try these! The oats will help support your mood and the peanut butter will give you the extra protein and fat you need during the luteal phase.

CHEWY PEANUT BUTTER COOKIES

Prep and cook time: 25 minutes
Makes: 10 cookies

What you need:

330g / 11½oz / 1½ cups smooth peanut butter (or almond or
   cashew)
100g / 3½oz / ½ cup coconut sugar (take this to about 50–70g /
   4–5 tbsp if you want a less sweet version, and use brown sugar
   if you don't have coconut sugar)
5 tbsp melted butter
3 medium eggs
2 tsp vanilla extract
¼ tsp bicarbonate of soda / baking soda
180g / 6¼oz oats (I used jumbo rolled oats, but regular pinhead /
   steel-cut would work too)

How to make it:

1. Preheat the oven to 160°C fan / 180°C / 350°F / gas
   mark 4.
2. Mix together the peanut butter, coconut sugar and
   melted butter until well combined.
3. Add the eggs, vanilla extract and baking soda and
   combine again, then gradually stir in the oats.
4. Line a baking sheet with parchment paper and use
   a tablespoon to spoon 10 cookies onto the paper,
   leaving a gap between each to allow the cookies to
   spread slightly while they cook.
5. Bake for 10 minutes or until the edges are golden
   brown. The middles should be slightly underdone –
   that's what makes them a little chewy!
6. Remove from the tray onto a wire rack to cool. Enjoy!

Improving Your Luteal Phase by Managing Your Energy Levels

It's natural for our energy levels to gradually decline as we move through the luteal phase and get closer and closer to our periods. There's a tendency to try to push through, with many of us often using coffee, tea and other caffeinated drinks to prop up our energy. Before you think I'm about to tell you to stop drinking coffee and tea entirely (I'm not going to do that!), I have to tell you about the major coffee habit I used to have. On an average working day, I'd drink between five and seven cups of black coffee. Hardcore, I know. I needed it to get me going in the morning, especially after a night that featured three to four glasses of red wine. My issues with alcohol could fill an entire book.

After a while, I began to make the link between how much coffee I was drinking, the tired and wired feelings, the sugar cravings, the anxiety I felt and some of the premenstrual symptoms I was experiencing. The research doesn't currently show any connection between caffeine and premenstrual symptoms; however, we do know that caffeine does increase cortisol levels.[46] High cortisol levels can lead to energy crashes, sugar cravings, mood changes and increased inflammation, all of which can worsen premenstrual symptoms. Some of us may also have premenstrual insomnia and too much caffeine, especially after 2pm, can make this worse.

If you find yourself relying on coffee, tea and other caffeinated drinks and you'd like to cut down, here are a few things you can try:

- Limit your coffee or tea to the morning
- Drink one to two cups only and really enjoy the ritual of making and drinking each cup
- Drink your coffee or tea in smaller cups
- Drink your coffee with your breakfast and / or your morning snack to help slow the effects of the caffeine on cortisol and blood sugar

- Swap to green tea or matcha, a powdered green tea
  The caffeine in green tea is broken down much slower
  in the body, reducing the caffeine jitters. You also get
  the benefits of l-theanine, an amino acid that increases
  the alpha waves in the brain, which calms us and
  increases concentration

Improving Your Luteal Phase With Exercise and Movement

As we talked about in the last section, our energy levels
gradually decline as we go through our luteal phase. When I
talk about exercise, many women have shared that they've
felt really down on themselves when they can't exercise with
the same intensity throughout their menstrual cycle.

My advice is to embrace these changes and listen to your
body. You may lean into slower forms of exercise such as
swimming, slow flow yoga, a long walk or hike or a bike ride.
The rise of progesterone after ovulation means we have
slightly less glucose available, so the endurance exercise you
do during ovulation may still feel good for you during the
early stages of the luteal phase. Instead of pushing through,
take it day by day and move your body in a way that feels
right to you. That might be a lower-intensity version of what
you normally do.

A Few Yoga Poses for the Luteal Phase

When we get to our late luteal phase, we may feel called to
move a little slower and away from our regular high-energy
workouts. Embrace this feeling by adding in yoga poses that
are centred on rest and focusing on the breath – your inhale
and your exhale.

Corpse pose / *Shavasana*

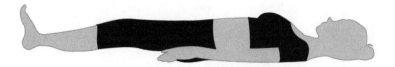

Shavasana may be one of the most challenging poses because it asks us to embrace stillness and focus on our breath. In *shavasana*, close your eyes, take up space, spreading your arms and legs out wide and bring your attention to the space in between your eyes to help focus the mind. If you find your attention wandering, know that this is normal. Acknowledge the thoughts that are coming in and let them drift away, bringing your focus back to your breath. If possible, stay in *shavasana* for a few minutes or longer, allowing yourself this time to just be.

Child's pose / *Balasana*

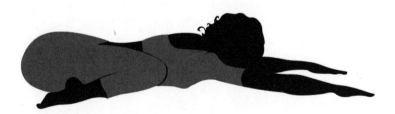

This is another very restful pose that asks us to bring our attention to our breath and slow down. You have several options with your arms in this pose; they can be stretched out in front or you can bring them behind you with your palms facing the sky. Stay in this pose as long as you like, enjoying the time to rest.

Puppy pose / *Uttana Shishosana*

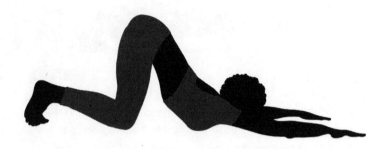

Puppy pose is a lovely alternative to child's pose that helps open up the shoulders and chest. With your arms stretched out in front of you, you have the option of keeping your head lifted to deepen the stretch in your chest or you can place your forehead onto the ground. Slow down and connect with your breath. You may stay in this pose for a minute or longer and then shift back to child's pose.

What You Can Try During the Luteal Phase

Here's a summary of the different recommendations in this chapter. Start by adding whatever resonates with you the most.

Food	Exercise / Movement
• Increase the amount of protein and healthy fats in your meals	• Listen to your body and do what feels right to you that day – don't force it!
• Tryptophan: poultry, red meat, pork, salmon, beans, pumpkin seeds, oats, eggs	• Endurance exercise such as long runs, cycles or swims in the early luteal phase when progesterone is still high
• Calcium: sardines, salmon, full-fat yogurt, whole milk, cheese, tahini, spinach, black-eyed beans / peas, almonds	**Lifestyle**
• Potassium: potatoes, apricots, prunes / dried plums, banana, artichokes, oranges, sunflower seeds, eggs	• Slow down as you get further into the luteal phase
	• Harness the "get sh*t done" energy, but don't feel like you have to do everything!
• Iodine: seaweed, cod, Jersey potatoes, prawns / shrimp, whole milk, eggs, tuna, strawberries	• Notice your mood and if any mood changes are the result of external events or if they're the result of hormonal changes

PART 3

Specific Conditions and Complaints

CHAPTER 8

'Why 'Is 'My 'Period So F***ing 'Painful? – 'Physical 'Problems and 'How to 'Relieve Them

Most of us have experienced at least one painful period and some of us have them every single menstrual cycle. Many will just grin and bear it, thinking it's a normal part of having a period. I definitely did! A study by the University of Birmingham in the UK[1] showed that 20 per cent of women studied experienced menstrual cramping severe enough to interfere with daily activities.

Speaking of grinning and bearing it, a 2017 Dutch study of over 30,000 women found that 80 per cent of the women studied continued to work and study while experiencing period pain and were less productive as a result.[2] It's not surprising, is it? It's hard to give your full focus to anything when you're dealing with what feels like a rebellious uterus. Research by the menstrual product brand Bodyform found persistent cultural and societal beliefs that bearing pain is considered the woman's role and that women need to "just get on with it".[3]

Think about it like this: on average, we may have between 9 and 15 periods every year.[4] If we experience two or three days of pain every period, that's up to 45 days of pain every year. Does that seem normal to you? Would we accept this in any other condition? I would like to think that the answer would be no.

Not all painful periods are created equal. Is your period pain bad? Sometimes, it can *just* be period pain (of course, I say *just* because pain is pain and even if it's not associated with another condition, it needs to be taken seriously). This type of period pain is known as primary dysmenorrhea and is typically caused by excessive uterine contraction caused by high numbers of prostaglandins, the hormone-like compounds that cause the uterus to contract in order to shed its lining.

And sometimes it can be something more. This is called secondary dysmenorrhea, when the pain you experience during your period is caused by another condition, such as endometriosis, adenomyosis, uterine fibroids or pelvic inflammatory disease (PID). Ovarian cysts and uterine polyps can also make periods more painful than they need to be.

In this chapter, we'll talk about what might be going on for you.

Nora's Story

When Nora first came to see me, she didn't pull any punches. She sat down in front of me and said, "Le'Nise, why is my period so f***ing painful?" Nora had been dealing with painful periods for most of her adult life, periods which had only become worse as she had grown older. She had been to see her doctor, who told her that periods were supposed to be painful, prescribed her strong painkillers and sent her on her way.

After trying these painkillers and finding they didn't really touch the sides of the period pain, she went back to her doctor, who said that she just needed to find a way to deal with the pain. Imagine (actually, I'm sure many of you don't need to imagine, as you've had a similar experience!) being told by a doctor that you just need to find a way to deal with pain. It's shocking – and it's something I hear a lot from clients.

But it's not true, and I really want you to hear and absorb this message. You don't need to just find a way to deal with your period pain. Period pain may be common, but it's not normal.

After trying to deal with the painful periods herself with hot water bottles and random supplements she found through Dr Google, Nora eventually found her way to my clinic. She described the nature of the period pain she was experiencing, and I was convinced that this wasn't just period pain and that she could potentially have endometriosis. I'll discuss endometriosis later in this chapter: the signs and symptoms, the different forms and what to do to manage and improve the pain that characterizes this condition.

I gave Nora a letter to take to her doctor explaining my endometriosis hypothesis and asked them to consider further investigation, including a transvaginal ultrasound, which can suggest the presence of ovarian endometriosis, ahead of a more invasive laparoscopy, a type of surgery that is currently the only definitive way to diagnose this condition. In the meantime, we started to work on Nora's diet, adding in more leafy green vegetables, cruciferous vegetables and other anti-inflammatory foods. I asked her to look at the amount of sugar, caffeine and alcohol she was consuming, explaining that, in excess, these could contribute to the inflammation that may have been driving her period pain.

We also looked at her gut health in order to support her immune system and reduce the digestive symptoms she experienced right before and during her period, including bloating and cycling between diarrhoea and constipation.

Throughout our time working together, I explained to Nora that the work we were doing on her diet and lifestyle wouldn't mean instantaneous changes to the period pain, but rather, her periods would become less painful over time and would hopefully become more manageable.

After six months of consistent changes to her diet, better sleep hygiene, incorporating more exercise, including yoga and working with a physiotherapist to work on pelvic alignment, Nora shared that her period pain had dramatically decreased, and she felt like she could live a normal life when she had her period and had a toolkit to deal with the pain if it did increase.

Painful Periods

Before we go any further, let's be clear on what we mean by pain. It's paramount that we have a vocabulary to describe the pain we experience. The International Association for the Study of Pain defines pain as "an unpleasant sensory and emotional experience associated with, or resembling that associated with, actual or potential tissue damage" and expands upon it with the following context:

- Pain is always a personal experience that is influenced to varying degrees by biological, psychological and social factors
- Pain and nociception (i.e. perception or sensation of pain) are different phenomena. Pain cannot be inferred solely from activity in sensory neurons
- Through their life experiences, individuals learn the concept of pain

- A person's report of an experience as pain should be respected
- Although pain usually serves an adaptive role, it may have adverse effects on function and social and psychological wellbeing
- Verbal description is only one of several behaviours to express pain; inability to communicate does not negate the possibility that a human or a nonhuman animal experiences pain[5]

Using this definition, when I discuss period pain in this chapter, I'm not referring to a few light cramps or twinges or a dull ache that passes quickly in the first few days of a period. To be clear, I'm not dismissing this pain, but this isn't the type of pain that is necessarily going to stop you in your tracks. What I'm referring to is pain that requires painkillers to keep you going, pain that requires you to completely change your daily schedule, pain that feels excessive and debilitating to you, pain that has an impact on your mental health, or pain that causes vomiting or diarrhoea.

Let's talk about five reasons that period pain might be happening.

1. Inflammation
2. Endometriosis
3. Adenomyosis
4. Fibroids
5. Ovarian cysts

Inflammation
Let's have a little recap on inflammation.

Acute inflammation: a short-term immune system process designed to help protect you from infections and disease and to heal the body from injury.[6] It's beneficial!

Chronic inflammation: this occurs when the immune system is still working to heal and protect, even when there is no infection or injury present. This is most typically caused by high levels of stress, lack of sleep and too much sugar, alcohol and processed foods in the daily diet. Chronic inflammation can lead to side effects such as increased pain levels, fatigue, depression, anxiety and digestive issues like diarrhoea and constipation.[7]

Why is chronic inflammation such an issue? The World Health Organization ranks the diseases that occur from chronic inflammation – such as strokes, diabetes, dementia and chronic respiratory illnesses – as the greatest threats to human health.[8]

Factors such as age, endocrine-disrupting chemicals (EDCs), obesity, a diet high in trans fats and sugar, chronic stress, chronic sleep issues, smoking and unbalanced sex hormones[9] increase the risk of chronic inflammation. What does this mean for us in our day-to-day lives? We're more stressed, we're trying to get by on less sleep, we're eating on the run, we're eating fewer fruits and vegetables and more of us are constipated, i.e. not having a daily bowel movement, all of which increase the risk of chronic inflammation.

A 2016 cross-section analysis by researchers at the University of California, Davis, suggests that period pain is caused by inflammation, measured by high levels of an inflammatory blood marker called C-reactive protein (CRP).[10] Researchers have also found that those with period pain have a higher number of prostaglandins,[11] hormone-like compounds typically associated with inflammation. They are also responsible for different functions in the body, including:

- Blood pressure
- Controlling blood flow
- Regulating body temperature
- Pain and fevers
- Blood clot formation and removal
- Breathing

- Digestion
- Regulating ovulation and menstruation

So not all prostaglandins are bad!

When it comes to periods, research has found that women with primary dysmenorrhea have elevated levels of a specific type of prostaglandin called PGF2α.[12, 13] These stimulate the muscular layer of the uterus, the myometrium, resulting in increased contractions and irregular rhythms. In other words, more of them make your periods more painful.

We must also remember that menstruation itself is an inflammatory process because the uterus produces prostaglandins to force the uterus to contract and shed its lining. The issue is that those with painful periods typically have more PGF2α, which makes periods more painful. Let's talk about how to reduce chronic inflammation.

How to Reduce Chronic Inflammation

If we consider what causes chronic inflammation – chronic stress, lack of sleep, an unbalanced diet and too much alcohol – there's a lot that we can do to reduce it.

Let's start with food.

What we eat three times a day, for breakfast, lunch and dinner, can have a powerful impact on our body's ability to reduce chronic inflammation. And we now know that by reducing chronically high levels of inflammation, we can reduce period pain.

As I've discussed throughout this book, in my clinical practice, I prefer to focus on adding in food, drink and herbs that are supportive for the body, rather than focusing on what needs to be removed. Eventually, I do have to have a conversation with some clients about the effects of sugar, chocolate, highly processed and packaged foods, alcohol, soft drinks and vegetable oils in excess. To be clear, one person's excess is another person's moderation. However,

I find that many of us generally have a sense of when we're overdoing the cake, cookies and crisps or when we're drinking too much alcohol.

What I love to do with my clients with period pain is start our work together by adding foods in and getting them to focus on what they *can* eat and drink, rather than what they can't. I love it when they add in a mix of the anti-inflammatory foods and herbs in the table below to every meal, alongside anti-inflammatory supplements, which we'll talk about later in the chapter. This list isn't exhaustive but it's a great menu to choose from when thinking about how to add these foods into your meals.

Anti-inflammatory Foods, Herbs and Teas

Foods	Herbs, Spices and Teas
Wild oily fish eaten maximum 3 times a week	Ginger
Seeds such as pumpkin, flax, sesame, sunflower, chia	Turmeric
Fruits such as berries, pineapple, peaches, apples, oranges, watermelon, avocado	Green tea and matcha
Leafy green vegetables such as kale, spinach, chard, callaloo, pak choi/bok choy, spring/collard greens	Cinnamon
Cruciferous vegetables such as broccoli, asparagus, cauliflower, Brussels sprouts, kohlrabi	Garlic
Algae	Black pepper
Olive oil, coconut oil, ghee, butter	Cayenne pepper
Tomatoes	Rosemary
Nuts such as almonds, cashews, walnuts, pistachios	Basil
Mushrooms	Dill
Free-range, organic meat: beef, lamb, chicken	Oregano
Wild seafood such as oysters, mussels and clams, eaten maximum 3 times a week	
Whole grains such as quinoa, buckwheat, millet	
Legumes and pulses such as kidney beans, chickpeas/garbanzo beans, lentils, black beans	
Free-range eggs (eat the yolks!)	

Adding in a range of these foods, herbs, spices and teas on a consistent basis can have a powerful effect on inflammation and reduce levels over time.

As we've talked about, it's not just about the food and supplements that get added into the diet, it's also about what gets taken out. For some people, sugar, alcohol, cow's-milk dairy and gluten can be highly inflammatory, so if period pain is a major issue for you, it can be beneficial to trial reducing or removing these foods from the diet, especially if it can be done in a way that doesn't lead to a restrictive mindset around food. If you have a history of disordered eating or eating disorders, please work with a specialized practitioner who can help you do this a non-triggering way.

With my clients that are experiencing chronic period pain, I ask them to keep a food diary and then work with them to trial two weeks with less of the inflammatory foods they're eating most frequently. Sugar and alcohol tend to be what we work on the most, as removing them can make a significant difference to period pain.

Try jotting down how much sugar and alcohol you're consuming. Then look at how you can gradually reduce these foods, consuming them in a mindful way and taking the time to enjoy each bite or sip – and stopping when you've had enough. It's definitely easier said than done, but I believe that mindful eating and drinking is like a muscle: if you do this consistently and with intention, it will grow stronger as time goes on.

Anti-inflammatory Supplements

Vitamin D, omega-3 fatty acids and magnesium, which we have discussed earlier in the book, are all very potent anti-inflammatories that are beneficial in supplement form to help reduce painful periods.

For painful periods, try taking a fish oil supplement with at least 1,000mg and a higher proportion of EPA to DHA. If you're on any type of blood-thinning medication, speak to your doctor before taking any omega-3 supplements.

If you're going to try magnesium, the type you take matters. Magnesium glycinate is a fantastic all-rounder and easily absorbed by the digestive system. Try taking a 240mg capsule of magnesium in the morning with your breakfast all throughout your menstrual cycle. You may also want to topically apply a magnesium spray on any areas that are painful, such as your abdomen, legs or back, as this will have more of a local effect.

Try taking a 100mg capsule of vitamin B6 on days when period pain is strongest and make sure your daily multivitamin has at least 25mg. Additional supplementation with vitamin B6 and magnesium is a good way to manage period pain, because vitamin B6 can stimulate cell membranes in transferring magnesium and increase the amount of magnesium available for muscle relaxation.[14]

For more information on these supplements, go to page 158 (vitamin D), page 91 (omega-3 fatty acids) and page 87 (magnesium).

N-Acetylcysteine (NAC)

A 2009 Italian study found that n-acetylcysteine (NAC) was beneficial for both reducing endometriosis pain and reducing the size of endometriomas (cystic lesions that stem from the disease process of endometriosis and sometimes referred to as chocolate cysts).[15] In the study of 92 Italian women, 47 took 600mg of NAC three times a day for three months. Within the NAC treated group, 24 cancelled scheduled laparoscopies due to cysts decreasing or disappearing and or relevant pain reduction.[16]

Cysteine is an amino acid that is the precursor to glutathione, our body's master antioxidant, and n-acetyl-cysteine is the supplement form of this amino acid. We can get cysteine from eating high-protein foods such as high-quality red meat, poultry and pork, seafood and fish, beans, pulses, oats, eggs and dairy. NAC is a powerful anti-inflammatory supplement and if you have endometriosis, this supplement can be a valuable part of your pain-management toolkit.

Try taking 600mg of NAC twice a day for six months to help rebuild your body's antioxidant stores, which can be depleted in those with endometriosis.

Instant(ish) Relief for Period Pain

But what about when you're right in the middle of a painful period and need some instant relief?

Here are a few things to try that aren't painkillers.

Magnesium

Magnesium, nature's relaxing mineral, can be helpful for reducing and managing period pain. Leafy greens and nuts and seeds are a great source of this mineral. I usually recommend that my clients use magnesium in a similar way to painkillers. Try taking two to three capsules of magnesium glycinate a few days before your period and then up to six 240mg capsules on day 1 and 2 of your period, or two capsules every three to four hours.

Zinc

A 2016 study looking at the effectiveness of zinc in reducing primary dysmenorrhea found that taking zinc[17] was effective in reducing period pain on a long-term basis. Zinc has a powerful anti-inflammatory effect and can significantly reduce prostaglandin levels. Free-range, organic red meat such as beef and lamb, pumpkin and sunflower seeds, oysters and other seafood, eggs (eat the yolks!) and ginger are fantastic food sources of zinc. Try taking up to 80mg of zinc picolinate or citrate per day for up to three months.

Cramp Bark

Cramp bark is a herb that's been used for a long time in herbal medicine and has anecdotally been shown to provide pain relief due to its antispasmodic nature. Basically, it acts like a muscle relaxant and that helps reduce the intensity of uterine contractions.[18] Try taking 1 teaspoon three times a day during the days you experience period pain.

CBD

I'm personally a huge fan of cannabidiol (CBD), one of the over 100 non-psychoactive compounds of the cannabis plant. Research in this area is still in its infancy due to huge variations in local laws regulating cannabis, but there is growing support for the use of CBD for reducing chronic pain.[19] CBD acts on the endocannabinoid system, our natural cannabis-producing system in the body, through receptors which are concentrated in the brain, immune, nervous and female reproductive system. CBD has also been found to have an anti-inflammatory effect,[20] which makes it promising for use with chronic period pain.

In the UK, the CBD market is growing, although it is not well regulated. Dr Dani Gordon, the author of the book *The CBD Bible* (2020), says that we should look for a full-spectrum CBD, which means it's been extracted from the whole plant. If you can't find that, she says that pure CBD is still beneficial. I highly recommend Dr Gordon's book if you want to learn more about CBD.

TENS Machine

A transcutaneous electrical nerve stimulation (TENS) machine is typically used in childbirth but can also be a brilliant way of managing period pain. It works by stimulating the skin and uses current at various pulse rates and intensities to provide pain relief. A systematic review found that patients had at least moderate relief when using a TENS machine for period pain, hypothesizing that TENS is thought to work by altering the body's ability to receive or perceive pain signals rather than by having a direct effect on the uterine contractions.[21]

Heat

When the period pain I experienced was at its worst, a hot bath or hot water bottle always seemed to provide some relief. I would lie in the bath for hours, constantly topping up the water. The water was so hot that I would feel lightheaded when I got out. One research study compared heat therapy with ibuprofen and found that using a heat patch that was at least 39°C (102.2°F) for 12 hours a day was as effective as taking 400mg of ibuprofen three times a day, while another study found that heat therapy was superior to ibuprofen.[22, 23]

If you like using heat as a way of managing period pain, try rotating between heat patches, hot water bottles and hot baths to reduce the likelihood of burn marks on the skin, something I see frequently with my endometriosis clients.

Endometriosis

Endometriosis is a condition that affects at least 1 in 10 women of menstruating age[24] and possibly even more, because it can take up to 7.5 years to diagnose, sometimes even as long as 11 years(!).[25] If that's not shocking enough, a 2016 Italian study showed that six out of ten endometriosis cases go undiagnosed,[26] which means that many live with the often incredibly painful symptoms of endometriosis and think they just need to soldier on. A 2012 Austrian study found that normalization of endometriosis symptoms and period pain by both patients and doctors contributed to several of the delays in diagnosis.[27]

In my clinic and on my podcast, I see this regularly: women expecting to live with the pain of endometriosis or receiving a very late-in-life diagnosis, having spent years trying to get answers.

This was the situation that Jasmin Harsono, a guest on my podcast, *Period Story*, faced. She said that when she got her first period, she "pretty much got the symptoms of heavy bleeds, chronic pain straight away, and I lived through that for years until I was in my late 20s. I couldn't go on the Pill or anything like that because it caused me severe migraines. I had to really go through this cycle every month. And I had very long periods. They would be around ten days of bleed, heavy bleeding. And I couldn't get any answers. I had tests done, and it was kind of like, this is what periods are like. That's what I was told. And I kept thinking, 'This is not it. This is not it.'"

Jasmin then had an incident where a cyst ruptured, which caused her to go to A&E. It was only then that she was finally diagnosed with endometriosis. She said that by that time, she understood and had a level of understanding that "my whole life, all these experiences with my period were because I had endometriosis. Then I had a link to that and the more knowledge I had, the more power I had and the less blame I had on my period. It was like, 'Oh, I actually had something wrong with me all this time. I had this condition.' And then I wanted to support myself in getting well. That's how it became full circle in the end."

The time from her first period to her endometriosis diagnosis was over 20 years.

In endometriosis, cells similar to those that normally stay in the lining of the womb are also found in different parts of the body, such as the abdomen, bowels, legs and sometimes even the brain, nose and lungs.[28]

This tissue becomes problematic during menstruation because it acts similarly to the tissue in the lining of the uterus, inflaming and attempting to shed. Because this tissue is outside the uterus, it has nowhere to go, which results in pain, additional inflammation and eventually scarring and creating adhesions, which can create even more problems.

There are four different stages of endometriosis,[29] based upon the location, depth and extent of the endometriosis implants (the endometrial tissues found outside the womb) and presence and size of endometrial implants in the ovaries. It's worth noting there are limits to defining endometriosis by its stage, as stage doesn't always correlate with the severity of the pain. I've seen clients who have stage IV endometriosis with relatively moderate pain and clients who have mild, stage II endometriosis with severe period pain.

Stage I: minimal, with small lesions or injuries and shallow endometrial implants on the ovaries, as well as some inflammation around the pelvis

Stage II: mild, with more lesions and implants on one or both ovaries and the pelvis

Stage III: moderate, with deeper implants on the ovaries and the pelvis and more lesions, some small endometriomas (also called chocolate cysts, because they're filled with old blood)

Stage IV: severe, with many deep implants on the pelvis and ovaries, extensive lesions on the fallopian tubes and bowels, large endometriomas on the ovaries

Endometriosis symptoms can vary widely in their intensity. They can include:

- Painful and / or heavy periods
- Constant tiredness
- Pelvic pain that worsens during menstruation
- Painful sex
- Painful urination and bowel movements
- Bloating (known as endo belly)
- Digestive symptoms such as cycling between constipation and diarrhoea
- Difficulty conceiving due to scar tissue on the womb, ovaries and fallopian tubes
- Depression

In moderate and severe endometriosis, there are also cysts, adhesions (areas of scar tissue that can cause organs or tissues to stick together) and more severe scarring. For some, excision surgery may be helpful, as this gives you the ability to start from scratch with your endometriosis management programme by removing endometriosis tissue. There are side effects to any surgical procedure, so please speak to your consultant or surgeon to see if this is a practical solution for you.

Managing inflammation, finding balance between oestrogen and progesterone and good gut health are important parts of managing the symptoms of endometriosis. As we discussed earlier in the chapter, pain is a symptom of inflammation, so where there is pain, there is always some degree of inflammation.

For anyone with endometriosis, addressing the symptoms of inflammation with the different tools we talked about earlier in the chapter will be helpful.

Let's talk about two other areas that need to be addressed in order to reduce and manage endometriosis pain.

Finding Balance Between Oestrogen and Progesterone

Until very recently, the symptoms of endometriosis were thought to be driven by excess oestrogen: levels of this hormone that are too high in relation to progesterone. We now know that endometriosis is primarily an issue of immune system dysregulation. However, addressing the symptoms of excess oestrogen and bringing oestrogen back in balance in relation to progesterone is key for managing endometriosis pain. In animal studies, it was found that high levels of oestrogen caused the uterus to contract more strongly by producing more prostaglandins. We can hypothesize this also contributes to stronger period pain.[30, 31]

When thinking about bringing oestrogen levels back into balance, it's important to address three areas: what you eat, what you put on your body and the health of your gut.

How the Type of Foods You Eat Support Oestrogen Balance

In Chapter 4, we talked about the different types of oestrogens in our body. We learned that what we eat helps our liver break down oestrogens to a less powerful form to then be eliminated by our bowels through our stool.

Let's get into this in more detail. Here's a little science for you: when our body is finished using the oestrogen that has either been created in the ovaries, adrenals (the small glands on our kidneys) and adipose tissue or has accumulated from external sources of oestrogen (xenoestrogens), such as from pesticides in foods, plastics, environmental pollution, synthetic chemicals in skincare, make-up, haircare and cleaning products,[32] it all needs to be broken down by the liver. Our liver breaks down these different forms of oestrogen in three phases, which is called detoxification. Here's a simple explanation:

Phase I: uses a family of liver enzymes called cytochromes P450 (CYP) to break down oestrogens produced by our body and xenoestrogens from a fat-soluble form to more potent water-soluble forms (2-OH, 4-OH and 16a-OH) so they can work with the liver enzymes needed in Phase II detoxification.[33]

Phase II: takes the oestrogens that have been broken down in Phase I and adds additional liver enzymes to neutralize them

Phase III: the products of Phase II detoxification are moved through the intestines with bile from the gallbladder and then excreted in one of three ways:

- via a bowel movement
- sent through the kidney and excreted through our urine
- through the skin via sweat

Daily bowel movements that are solid and easy to pass, regular trips to the loo to urinate and time to sweat a few times a week are the best ways to make sure this process of elimination happens!

When this process of detoxification isn't working well, such as when we're constipated, it impacts the amount of oestrogen in our bodies and can lead to us having too much.

This means oestrogen is not being effectively moved out the body through our bowel movements and will be recycled back into circulation. Our gut health and an enzyme called beta-glucuronidase also have an impact on this. I'll go into this later in the chapter.

What we eat and drink has a huge impact on the way the liver breaks down oestrogen.

The following tables contain the nutrients and foods we need to support the three phases of liver detoxification.[34, 35] You'll notice we talked about these foods in the last four chapters. How many of them are already in your daily meals?

Key Nutrients for Phase I Detoxification[36, 37]

Nutrient	Food
Vitamin A	Full-fat dairy, liver, eggs
Vitamin B1	Beef, nuts, oats, eggs, oranges, seeds, liver
Vitamin B2	Beef, dairy, eggs, mushrooms, wild salmon, liver, almonds
Vitamin B3	Red meat, oily fish and seafood, dark leafy greens, asparagus, avocados
Vitamin B6	Sweet potatoes, spinach, bananas, dark leafy greens, offal/organ meats, oily fish, sunflower seeds
Folate	Dark leafy greens, broccoli, beetroot/beet, cauliflower, lentils, asparagus
Vitamin B12	Red meat, full-fat dairy, eggs
Vitamin C	Citrus, berries, red, yellow and green peppers, broccoli, cauliflower, pineapple, mango
Vitamin E	Almonds, sunflower seeds, spinach, spring/collard greens
Beta-carotene	Carrots, sweet potatoes, leafy greens, broccoli, squash, tomatoes and most other fruits and vegetables with an orange, yellow or green colour
Magnesium	Dark leafy greens, nuts, seeds, pulses, seafood, avocados, bananas, cacao
Zinc	Red meat, seafood, pumpkin seeds, lentils, cashews, almonds
Selenium	Brazil nuts, sesame, flax, sunflower seeds, seafoods, offal/organ meats, mushrooms, beef, chicken

Key Foods for Phase II Detoxification

Dandelion	Oily fish
Citrus	Berries
Turmeric	Honeybush tea
Cruciferous vegetables such as kale, broccoli, watercress, pak choi/bok choy, Brussels sprouts, cauliflower	Brightly coloured fruits and vegetables
Onions, garlic, leeks, chives	Rosemary

How Our Gut Health Supports Oestrogen Balance

I'm fascinated by the power of our guts. When we talk about our gut and gut health, what we're referring to is our large and small intestines, which are in the area that most of us call our bellies or tummies.

Research has established a strong link between gut health and immune, mental and overall digestive health. Did you know that there's also a connection between our gut health and our hormone health? Regulation of oestrogen levels is largely dependent on our gut health and the health of our gut microbiome: the diverse array of bacteria, virus, fungi and protozoans that live in our small and large intestines.

It gets even better. We have a group of special bacteria and other microbes whose genes give them the ability to metabolize oestrogens.[38] In other words, we have microbes in our gut to help break oestrogen down, which we call the estrobolome. The estrobolome also impacts the way oestrogen is broken down by regulating the way it circulates around and out of the body.[39]

Our gut bacteria also produce an enzyme called beta-glucuronidase. We want to make sure we have low levels of this enzyme. When beta-glucuronidase is too high, it can reverse the process of breaking down oestrogens and reactivate them back into circulation in the body, leading to excess oestrogen and potentially, more period pain.[40]

In a nutshell, good gut health will have a powerful hormone-balancing effect in cases of the excess oestrogen that we can see in endometriosis. The bacterial composition of the estrobolome will be affected by age, ethnicity, diet, alcohol and antibiotic use. However, what we eat and drink can make positive changes to this part of our gut microbiome. This will then have a positive effect on the balance between oestrogen and progesterone in our body and reduce levels of beta-glucuronidase.[41]

There are several ways we can use food to support good gut health and a healthy estrobolome.

Increase Fibre

An easy way to add more fibre into your meals is to increase the number of vegetables on your plate, especially leafy green and cruciferous vegetables. Studies show that a diet rich in plant-based fibres can bring down beta-glucuronidase levels and support healthy oestrogen metabolism.[42] I will typically suggest that my clients make at least 50 per cent of their meal vegetable-based. If that sounds challenging, try adding one new vegetable each week in a variety of colours. Try adding the fruits and vegetables in the Eat The Rainbow Challenge in the table opposite if you fancy trying it for yourself!

Add Prebiotic and Probiotic Foods

Remember the analogy of the garden to describe how we should support our gut microbiome? Prebiotics are like the fertilizer of the garden (your gut microbiome) – these foods help the garden grow and stimulate the growth of healthy bacteria in the gut. Essentially, they are highly fibrous foods that provide fuel for the bacteria in the gut.[43]

The seeds of the garden are probiotic foods which bring new types of bacteria to your gut microbiome. These are typically aged, fermented foods and drinks that already have different strains of bacteria in them.[44]

Eat the Rainbow Challenge

Green	**Red**	**Yellow / Orange**	**Blue / Purple**	**Brown / White**
Spinach	Red Pepper	Carrots	Beetroot/Beets	Cauliflower
Kale	Radishes	Yellow Carrots	Purple Cabbage	Brown Pears
Asparagus	Radicchio	Sweet Potato	Aubergine/	Mushrooms
Broccoli	Red Onion	Pumpkin	Eggplant	White Peaches
Peas	Red Cabbage	Sweetcorn	Purple	Garlic
Green Beans	Red Chillies	Squash	Sprouting	Onions
Lettuce	Red Leaf	Yellow	Broccoli	Shallots
Cabbage	Lettuce	Courgettes/	Purple Carrots	Parsnips
Celery	Red Potatoes	Zucchini	Purple Sweet	Trunips
Cucumber	Red Carrots	Golden	Potatoes	Celeriac
Green Pepper	Rhubarb	Beetroot/Beets	Ocha/Oca	Potatoes
Watercress	Ocha/Oca	Yellow Pepper	Purple Endives	Jerusalem
Swiss Chard	Tomatoes	Orange Pepper	Purple	Artichokes
Parsley	Strawberries	Tumeric	Cauliflower	Spring Onions/
Coriander	Cherries	Ginger	Blackberries	Scallions
Mint	Red Grapes	Yellow	Blueberries	Leeks
Dill	Raspberries	Tomatoes	Purple Grapes	Dates
Rocket	Watermelon	Peaches	Plums	Coconut
Pak Choi/Bok	Red Apples	Nectarines	Figs	Lychees
Choy	Blood Oranges	Apricots	Blackcurrants	
Spring/Collard	Pink Grapefruit	Grapefruit	Prunes	
Greens	Red Pears	Rockmelon	Elderberries	
Brussel Sprouts	Pomegranate	Lemons		
Globe	Cranberries	Pineapples		
Artichokes	Redcurrants	Mangoes		
Samphire		Oranges		
Turnip Greens		Yellow		
Beet Greens		Watermelon		
Courgettes/		Cataloupe		
Zucchini		Papaya		
Sugar Snaps		Persimmons		
Mange Tout		Tangerines		
Romanesco		Clementine		
Cauliflower		Physalis		
Green Apples		Bananas		
Green Grapes		Plantains		
Limes				
Kiwifruit				
Pears				
Honeydew				
Melon				
Avocados				

Here's a list of these two types of foods you can try to add into your meals.

Probiotic Food and Drink	Prebiotic Foods
Kombucha	Onions
Kimchi	Garlic
Sauerkraut	Jerusalem artichoke
Pickled vegetables	Unripened bananas
Kvass	Artichokes
Kefir	Chicory/endive root
Full-fat plain yogurt	Dandelion greens
Miso	Leeks
Fermented tofu	Oats
Natto	Apples
Tempeh	Cocoa
Buttermilk	Seaweed
Some aged cheeses like Asiago, Stilton, Cheddar, Gouda	Flaxseed

Take Probiotics With Specific Strains of Bacteria

A 2008 randomized controlled trial found that prebiotics, as well as certain strains of bacteria, had a positive effect on reducing beta-glucuronidase levels.[45] The study found that the prebiotics lactulose and inulin and the probiotic L. casei Shirota all resulted in decreased beta-glucuronidase.

Try to find probiotics with this strain, rather than taking any brand of probiotic available.

Please find additional endometriosis resources at the end of this book.

Adenomyosis

Adenomyosis is commonly misdiagnosed as endometriosis, because the symptoms can appear quite similar, until further examination. Adenomyosis is a condition where some of the tissue that normally grows in the lining of the uterus grows in the muscular wall of the uterus (the myometrium) instead.[46]

According to the NHS, around one in ten women will have adenomyosis.[47] This condition can occur in anyone who still has periods but is most common in women aged 40 to 50 and in women who have had children. Many with adenomyosis will often also have endometriosis, and diagnosis can be challenging, which is why this condition is often misdiagnosed or underdiagnosed.[48]

Adenomyosis can be an incredibly painful condition because the endometrial tissue continues to act as it normally does – thickening during the follicular phase of the menstrual cycle and breaking down and bleeding during the menstrual phase, without anywhere to shed. This can lead to an enlarged uterus. If there are high levels of inflammation in the body, this can also lead to painful and heavy periods for some, while others only experience slight discomfort. The heavy periods that are part of this condition can also lead to iron-deficiency anaemia, because too much iron has been lost through menstrual blood.

Another challenging part of living with adenomyosis is the pelvic pain and discomfort in the pelvis some experience during the seven to ten days before they get their period.[49]

Adenomyosis is typically characterized by the extreme pain that happens right before and during menstruation. Chronic inflammation and high prostaglandin levels can increase pain, so, as with endometriosis, managing this is important for reducing the symptoms of adenomyosis.

Please refer to the earlier sections on inflammation, reducing excess oestrogen and supporting gut health, as all these are also beneficial for managing pain in adenomyosis.

Please find additional adenomyosis resources at the end of this book.

Fibroids

Uterine fibroids are benign, non-cancerous growths that develop in, on or within the muscular lining of the uterus. They are the most common condition affecting the female reproductive system in the UK.[50] Fibroids are also known as uterine myomas, fibromyomas or leiomyomas. Fibroids can decrease and increase in size or even gradually disappear.

There are four main types of fibroids:[51]

1. **Intramural:** the fibroid is within the muscular uterine wall
2. **Submucosal:** the fibroid bulges into the uterine cavity, distorts the endometrium or is below the mucosal surface. Additionally, there are three types of submucosal fibroids:
   - Type 0: contained entirely within the endometrial cavity
   - Type 1: at least 50 per cent of the fibroid is in the endometrial cavity
   - Type 2: a fibroid that intrudes into the endometrial cavity, but at least 50 per cent of its bulk is within the uterine wall
3. **Subserosal:** the fibroid projects or protrudes to the outside of the uterus, giving the uterus an irregular shape
4. **Pedunculated:** the fibroid has a small stalk connecting it to the uterus

They can affect many women, sometimes with no symptoms at all. However, studies show that women of African origin or ancestry are more likely to develop fibroids that are significantly larger, grow for longer and faster and have more severe symptoms.[52] African ancestry is considered a significant risk factor for fibroids.[53]

A 2003 American study found that 80 per cent of the Black women studied had developed fibroids before the age of 50, compared to 70 per cent of white women.[54] Very little is currently understood about why fibroids disproportionately affect Black women; however, this study demonstrates that fibroids are much more common that we realize.

Although one of the main symptoms of fibroids is heavy menstrual bleeding, pelvic pain and period pain are also major symptoms. We don't know much about why fibroids start to grow, although a genetic link has been hypothesized. There are many families where women in every generation are affected by fibroids inherited from both the maternal and paternal line.

What we do know is that excess oestrogen in the body causes fibroids to grow.

There is also increased risk from diet, smoking and xenoestrogens from environmental pollutants, haircare and skincare products, such as relaxers, make-up, cleaning products and non-organic menstrual products, which increase the toxin burden on the liver and add to the work that it needs to do to break down oestrogens and clear them from the body. For a refresher on this, see page 223.

Low vitamin D status,[55] which tends to be more common among people with darker skin, also increases fibroid risk. Although there is not enough evidence to make a direct link, we can address vitamin D levels as part of a holistic programme to prevent further fibroid growth. See page 158 for specific actions to improve vitamin D status.

In my work with clients with fibroids, rebalancing oestrogen levels and reducing xenoestrogens has always been a major focus. Once this is under control, I find that my clients will typically have reduced symptoms from their fibroids, which often stop growing.

Thyroid health is an area that has been overlooked in fibroid management. The health of the thyroid is impacted by, and will impact, oestrogen levels in the body, and we know that fibroid growth is driven by excess oestrogen. If you have fibroids, I strongly recommend having your thyroid levels checked, so that you can manage the fibroids in a truly holistic way. For more information about which tests to ask your doctor for, go to Chapter 3.

When I was growing up, my mother had fibroids and suffered from heavy, painful and long periods. It was her experience, as I discussed in the introduction to this book, that made me think for years that this was a normal way to have a period. She eventually went on to have a partial hysterectomy, in which her uterus was removed, along with two grapefruit-size fibroids.

Shockingly, hysterectomy remains the most common treatment for fibroids,[56] although there are other less invasive treatments emerging, including:

- **Myomectomy:** surgical removal of the fibroid
- **Uterine fibroid embolization (UFE):** small particles are injected that cut off the blood flow to the fibroids
- **Myolysis:** a laser or electric current destroys the fibroids and shrinks the blood vessels that feed them
- **Cryomyolysis:** freezes the fibroids

Please find additional fibroids resources at the end of this book.

Ovarian Cysts

An ovarian cyst is a fluid-filled sac that develops on or in the ovary.[57] In most cases, we can have cysts on our ovaries, and they don't cause us any problems. It's only when they are too large, in the wrong place, or burst, that we feel the negative effects of ovarian cysts, including painful periods, painful ovulation, bloating, mid-cycle spotting and painful urination and / or bowel movements.

There are a few types of ovarian cysts:[58]

- **Follicular cysts:** These are the result of incomplete ovulation when the follicle doesn't open and release the mature egg cell. The follicle gradually becomes filled with fluid and can turn into a cyst

- **Corpus luteum cysts:** These occur when a corpus luteum continues to grow, rather than break down when it has finished releasing oestrogen and progesterone. It then fills with blood and / or fluid
- **Ovarian endometriomas (chocolate cysts):** These are cysts within the ovary that fill with old, dark blood and are associated with a more severe form of endometriosis

Some cysts can develop and go away on their own. In the case of polycystic ovarian syndrome (PCOS), I often see women who have been diagnosed with PCOS because of cysts appearing on an ultrasound, but when they have blood or urine testing to see what's happening on a hormonal level, the results don't often indicate PCOS. As we'll discuss in Chapter 10, you can have polycystic ovaries (PCO) without having PCOS and you can have PCOS without having PCO.

Supporting a healthy balance between oestrogen and progesterone is the best way to reduce ovarian cysts (see page 222). This balance helps follicles develop into healthy eggs that are released during ovulation and a corpus luteum that releases enough progesterone (and oestrogen) and breaks down as it should once it has fulfilled its purpose.

Tracking Your Pain

We know that some periods can be painful and that you'll need to speak to your doctor or another healthcare professional about the pain, especially if it regularly goes beyond a few aches and twinges.

To have a productive conversation, it's important to track your pain over at least three menstrual cycles and qualify it. As I discussed earlier, this helps give us a vocabulary to describe the pain we experience.

First, start to track when the pain happens during each period. Give the pain a number: 1 would be a gentle twinge, 10 would be pain that leaves you bed bound and unable to move. Then rank the pain: is it mild, moderate or severe? How often does it happen? What kind of pain is it: dull, throbbing, sharp, burning?

Then look at what else is going on in your life. What have you been eating? How stressed have you been? How much alcohol have you been drinking? Gather at least three months' worth of information so you can understand what normal is for you and what you can change about your lifestyle and what you eat, using the tools in this chapter, to help reduce your pain.

Your period and menstrual cycle are one of your body's vital signs, so if there's something persistently wrong with this vital sign, track and take note of what's happening for you so that you can get the appropriate support.

Take the following information to your doctor or healthcare professional:

- Size and location of the fibroids, if you have them
- A list of your symptoms
- Any medications or supplements you're taking

Also take a list of questions you would like them to answer such as:

- Potential routes to diagnosis, i.e. physical examinations, ultrasounds, blood, urine and stool tests
- A potential treatment plan
- Any potential referrals to specialists or consultants, and a timeline for this

Take notes during the consultation and ask for clarification when you're not sure what the doctor is saying. You can also ask if you can record the conversation. If you don't feel you can do this for yourself, bring someone with you that can help you advocate on your behalf.

Period Pain Tracker

	Cycle 1	Cycle 2	Cycle 3
When during your period is the pain happening?			
Rate the pain from 1 to 10			
Where is the pain happening?			
Rank the pain (mild, moderate, severe)			
How often does it happen?			
What kind of pain is it? Dull, throbbing, sharp, burning?			
What have you been doing to manage the pain?			

At the end of the appointment, ask for a copy of your medical report and any results from ultrasounds or physical exams. If you are refused any medication, blood tests or other examinations, ask for this refusal to be noted on your file so that you can refer back to it in the future.

You know your body best, so if you feel something is wrong, keep pushing until you get the answers and treatment you need and deserve.

For far too long, we've been told that period pain is a normal part of having a period. It is common, but it's not normal, and you don't need to grin and bear it anymore.

CHAPTER 9

'Why Am I So Moody? – Emotional Problems and How to Relieve Them

Moods and emotions are what make us human. It's normal to feel changes in your emotions over the course of each day, week, month and year. It's normal to have an emotional response to our thoughts and actions, as well as to external events. Aristotle, the Greek philosopher, argued that there were 14 distinct emotional expressions: anger, calm, confidence, contempt, emulation, enmity, envy, fear, friendship, indignation, kindness, pity, shame and shamelessness.

More recently, researchers at the University of Berkeley, California, have found that there are 27 distinct categories of emotion:[1]

- Admiration
- Adoration
- Aesthetic appreciation
- Amusement
- Anxiety
- Awe

- Awkwardness
- Boredom
- Calmness
- Confusion
- Craving
- Disgust

- Empathetic pain
- Entrancement
- Envy
- Excitement
- Fear
- Horror
- Interest
- Joy

- Nostalgia
- Romance
- Sadness
- Satisfaction
- Sexual desire
- Sympathy
- Triumph

And within each emotion, there can be so much nuance. Amusement can be a wry smile, a loud guffaw and somewhere in between.

This exploration of emotions shows that every day, we can cycle through a huge range of them. They can connect us with others and with our own thoughts, desires and experiences. Thinking about premenstrual mood changes, I believe that sometimes we can be too quick to write these off as simply part of PMS. I'd like us to remember that we're allowed to feel what we feel during every part of our cycle, and our feelings and emotions aren't lessened or invalidated because we experience them right before our period.

To reiterate what Dr Julie Holland said in her book *Moody Bitches*, oestrogen creates a veil of accommodation.[2] When oestrogen drops right before our period, our tolerance levels decline and we're less likely to put up with anything we've been accommodating during the rest of our menstrual cycle. As we explore the mood changes that some of us can experience in the second half of our menstrual cycle, I'd like to invite you to consider whether there have been times that you've been too quick to dismiss how you feel as PMS.

PMDD

Imagine this: for two weeks every month, a black cloud descends on you. You're exhausted, cartwheeling from anger to weepiness and back again. There are some days when you don't know how you can go on. You've never admitted that to anyone because it's scary to acknowledge that you've had such dark thoughts, but it's comforting to know that you might have a way out.

You've taken so much time off work, you're worried about losing your job. Your partner walks on eggshells around you, not knowing what mood they'll meet you in when they walk through the door. The doctor said it's just PMS, but you're not so sure about that. Your friends get PMS, and they just load up on chocolate and get a bit teary during *EastEnders*. You really don't know what to do.

This is the reality of PMDD. Premenstrual dysphoric disorder, or PMDD, affects 5 to 8 per cent of menstruating women,[3] across all races and ethnicities. We don't exactly know what causes PMDD, but there are a few theories. It's been hypothesized that a history of interpersonal trauma and post-traumatic stress disorder (PTSD)[4] can be risk factors for the onset of PMDD. We also know that there is a genetic aspect to PMDD, which means that it can run in families.

We must be clear that PMDD is not a more severe form of PMS. There may be some overlap in symptoms, but the biological mechanisms between the two are markedly different.

Remember the rise of progesterone and the second, smaller peak of oestrogen that occurs after ovulation? Ordinarily, these hormonal changes lead to a positive time in our menstrual cycle, with calm, settled moods and sustained energy. It's different for those with PMDD, who have a genetic susceptibility to be more sensitive and more negatively affected by the post-ovulatory rise in hormones.[5]

Some studies have found that women with PMDD have lower levels of cortisol and endorphins during the follicular phase, when we would expect them to be higher.[6] This suggests that there may be an issue with the HPA (hypothalamus–pituitary–adrenal) axis, the signalling pathway from our brain to our adrenal glands, the organs that produce cortisol and sit on top of our kidneys.

Additionally, some research has found that women with PMDD may have impaired functioning of allopregnanolone, a hormone metabolite created from progesterone and GABA, the brain neurotransmitter that helps calm us after ovulation.[7] Usually, allopregnanolone and GABA help settle the HPA axis. However, in those with PMDD, there is increased sensitivity to stress and anxiety after ovulation and during the luteal phase.

An easy way to summarize PMDD is to think of it as a cyclical mood disorder that causes an unwelcome post-ovulatory sensitivity to oestrogen, progesterone, allopregnanolone and GABA and a heightened post-ovulatory stress response.

PMDD is now listed in the Diagnostic and Statistical Manual of Mental Disorders, 5th Edition (DSM-5). If you're not familiar with the DSM-5, it's a manual that's used internationally to provide practitioners and doctors with standard language and diagnosis criteria for mental health disorders. The inclusion of PMDD in the DSM-5 means that a diagnosis is likely to happen more easily and you're more likely to be taken seriously when you approach your doctor about your symptoms.

Some of the core symptoms of PMDD can overlap with mood disorders and include:[8]

- Anxiety
- Irritability and anger
- Frequent mood changes
- Difficulty concentrating
- Feelings of worthlessness and hopelessness

There are some additional physical symptoms, including:

- Bloating
- Muscle pain and aches
- Breast tenderness

- Lethargy
- Appetite changes
- Sleep difficulties

At its most extreme, PMDD can manifest in suicidal ideation for some, which can be alarming and isolating. If you have experienced or are experiencing suicidal thoughts, please know that you're not alone and there is a lot of help out there. In the UK, the Samaritans are available 24/7 at samaritans.org or 116 123 or if you're in the US call 1 (800) 273-TALK.

For PMDD to be diagnosed, over the course of at least two to three consecutive menstrual cycles, you must have experienced five of the following symptoms from the final week before menstruation to within a few days of the next period.[9]

- Mood swings, feeling suddenly sad or tearful, increased sensitivity to rejection
- Irritability, anger or increased interpersonal conflict
- Markedly depressed mood, feelings of hopelessness or self-critical thoughts
- Notable anxiety, tension and / or feelings of being on edge

One of the following symptoms must also be present to reach a total of five symptoms:

- Decreased interest in usual activities
- Difficulty concentrating
- Lethargy, getting tired easily, notable lack of energy
- Notable lack of appetite, overeating or specific food cravings
- Sleep changes such as insomnia or hypersomnia (sleeping much more than usual)
- Feeling overwhelmed or out of control
- Physical symptoms such as breast tenderness / swelling, joint or muscle pain, bloating

The timing of the onset of PMDD symptoms is what distinguishes it from other mood disorders and other conditions.[10] These symptoms typically start after ovulation and dissipate after the start of the next period. They're usually very distressing, interfering with school, work, social activities and personal relationships.

Amara's Story

It was hard for Amara to pinpoint when the PMDD started for her, but once it hit, it took over her life. She said that she had one normal week every month: the rest were either dominated by PMDD symptoms or her period.

Her boyfriend called her Amara and Hyde, and she couldn't even be mad because she knew it was true. After ovulation, she turned into a different person. She would snap for no reason, flying into uncontrollable rages one minute and then collapsing into a heap of tears the next. The hardest part was knowing that she was behaving completely irrationally, and not being able to do anything about it.

Amara felt out of control. She'd been given a written warning for shouting at a client and knew she was on her last chance at work. Her boyfriend Steven was supportive and knew she didn't really mean it when she said hurtful things during her Hyde time. She didn't want to keep being so awful to him.

When I met Amara, she had just begun trying to find some answers. I encouraged her to go to her doctor with a list of her symptoms and the timings so that she could get a formal diagnosis of what we thought might be PMDD. In the meantime, I focused on nutritional and lifestyle support to make the time after ovulation easier for her.

We started by looking at her habits and routines. Amara wanted to have non-negotiables in place she could stick to even when the PMDD lethargy hit. I asked her to start batch cooking and freezing extra portions, so that she always had healthy options that she could defrost when she wasn't feeling great.

We also started adding in foods with nutrients that would help stabilize her moods and support her stress response after ovulation. I asked her to increase magnesium-rich foods such as pumpkin seeds, dark leafy greens like kale, chard, spinach and greens, hemp seeds, quinoa and Brazil nuts. The additional benefit of these foods are that they would help Amara rebalance oestrogen and overly high histamine levels, which may have been contributing to some of her PMDD symptoms, like bloating. For more about histamine and its impact on our hormone health, turn back to Chapter 6.

A small research study found that the addition of vitamin B6 through food and supplementation can help reduce PMDD symptoms,[11] so we increased the amount of vitamin B6 foods in Amara's meals to support oestrogen detoxification and to help stabilize the GABA receptors. This would help her not be so destabilized by the post-ovulatory rise in progesterone. Research shows that even mild vitamin B6 deficiency can downregulate GABA production,[12] so we added in vitamin B6 foods such as avocado, spinach, carrots, eggs, chickpeas/garbanzo beans, wild salmon and organic chicken and turkey, as well a good multivitamin with at least 25mg of B6. I asked Amara to reduce the amount of alcohol she was drinking, as it can deplete vitamin B6 levels.

Additionally, I asked Amara to take 480mg of magnesium glycinate each day for further mood and stress support. Because Amara's stress response was increased in the second half of her menstrual cycle, we looked at ways she could proactively manage stress and better identify and cope with her changing moods post-ovulation. This included getting a referral for cognitive behavioural therapy (CBT) from her doctor. The benefits of CBT for PMDD are backed by research. A 2019 study found that CBT was effective in addressing coping styles and integrating new ways of managing stress.[13]

Amara told me that for the first time, she felt hopeful about her future and her ability to cope with the PMDD symptoms.

Addressing PMDD Symptoms Through Food and Lifestyle Changes

If we think of PMDD as a cyclical mood disorder that causes: 1) an unfavourable post-ovulatory sensitivity to oestrogen, progesterone, allopregnanolone and GABA and 2) a heightened post-ovulatory stress response, then we need to make sure that we're doing what we can through food, lifestyle changes and stress reduction techniques to help mitigate these post-ovulatory physical and emotional changes.

Magnesium and B6

In Amara's story, we talked about the benefits of magnesium and B6 for reducing and managing PMDD symptoms. It's critical that you're including a wide variety of these foods in your meals every day. I also typically recommend that my clients with PMDD take a magnesium supplement and a multivitamin with vitamin B6 for at least three months. There may be an additional need for extra vitamin B6, but I don't usually go higher than 100mg for longer than six months, due to potential issues with nerve damage from high doses of B6.

Magnesium and B6 are also beneficial for supporting oestrogen metabolism, which is necessary so you don't go into ovulation with higher-than-normal levels of oestrogen, which can exacerbate mood-based PMDD symptoms. For more detail about foods that support oestrogen metabolism, flip back to Chapter 8.

Tryptophan Foods (and Gut Support!)

Although we expect serotonin levels to still be fairly high after ovulation, there is a hypothesis that those with PMDD may be more sensitive to the effects of oestrogen on serotonin function.[14] This can become more evident in the late luteal phase as serotonin levels decline alongside oestrogen.

Adding in tryptophan foods, like we discussed in Chapter 7, can be helpful for raising decreased late-luteal tryptophan levels and consequently, increasing serotonin levels. High protein foods such as free-range, organic red meat, eggs, cheese and poultry, wild salmon, fermented tofu, beans and seeds are a great way to increase your levels of this essential amino acid. Interestingly, pineapples, persimmons and bananas are also great ways to get tryptophan into your meals. They're all high in tryptophan and they're made up of simple carbohydrates, which, when eaten, force your body to release insulin from the pancreas. This then helps the body absorb more tryptophan.[15]

Don't forget that you make most of your serotonin in your gut. Keeping your gut healthy with regular bowel movements, fibre, fermented food and breaks between meals to give your body time to digest is important for making sure that you're continuing to make enough serotonin.

CBT

On the last page, we talked about the benefits of cognitive behavioural therapy (CBT) for PMDD. This type of therapy can be helpful because it gives you the tools to better identify when you're experiencing anger, irritability, mood swings and more. You also leave each session with actionable techniques you can use to cope with mood changes. For example, you'll be able to identify thought patterns and situations that act as triggers. Your therapist may ask you to start to note down these situations, the specific triggers and how you respond. They will then give you detailed techniques, coping thoughts, problem-solving and relaxation strategies you can use to respond differently.

A Mindful Moment

When I've talked about meditation before in this book, I've said that you don't need to force it if it doesn't work for you. Mindfulness, by way of focusing on a single task or activity, can help focus the mind into the present moment and away from anxious or unhelpful thoughts. Anything that requires you to be present can be mindful: cooking, baking, ironing, cleaning, sewing, knitting, painting, swimming, cycling, running or walking (without music or podcasts!). When you're really into these tasks and activities, you get into a state of flow. The psychologist Mihaly Csikszentmihalyi, who was the first to identify and research flow, says this means there is complete concentration on the task, in which time seems to either slow down or speed up, there is an effortlessness and ease, and the experience is intrinsically rewarding.[16] In a flow state, there is a loss of reflective self-awareness that can help those with PMDD get out of their own heads.

Exercise and Sleep

Exercise can be helpful in managing the mood-based symptoms of PMDD. Yoga is a lovely option because the combination of physical movement and breathwork is supportive of the nervous system, helping to reduce the stress response. And different types of yoga will have different benefits. A practice such as *ashtanga* or dynamic *vinyasa* flow puts more of a focus on *asana*, the physical part of yoga. This helps release endorphins and improve mood. Other forms of yoga – like *yin*, *Sivananda*, restorative or *Kundalini* – focus on moving energy around the body and *pranayama*, or breathwork, which provides additional support for the nervous system and can reduce the post-ovulatory stress response.

Sleep must be the foundation of your PMDD treatment strategy, especially during the first half of your menstrual cycle. Establishing good sleep habits can help reduce any post-ovulatory sleep disturbances.

Here are some examples of sleep habits you can start to add in:

- Expose your eyes to daylight first thing in the morning to help set your circadian rhythm (your body clock) so your brain understands it's daytime
- Limit caffeine to the morning, especially if you metabolize caffeine slowly
- Minimize screens at night. If you do use screens, use blue-light-blocking glasses to help your body produce more melatonin, the hormone that helps us get to sleep and stay asleep
- Create a bedtime routine for yourself that helps your body realize it's time to start to wind down, physically and mentally
- Sleep in a dark, quiet and cool room (I love using a sleep mask)
- Go to bed around the same time each night (ideally before 10.30pm)
- Wake up around the same time each morning

Other Treatment Options

A very small American study found that women with PMDD who were given the GnRH-releasing agonist leuprolide acetate (a drug that suppresses ovulation and the post-ovulatory release of oestrogen and progesterone) had a significant decrease in their symptoms.[17] For some of you, this may be the solution you are looking for. In the long term, though, it's worth considering the effects of the extended suppression of ovulation and loss of the benefits of progesterone, as these treatments reduce PMDD symptoms by creating a temporary, chemically induced menopause.

Others have had success using selective serotonin reuptake inhibitors (SSRIs) such as fluoxetine to manage PMDD symptoms. Please speak to your doctor to understand whether these would be right for you, including a discussion of the potential side effects and treatment time.

If you have PMDD, please know that you're not alone and there is a light at the end of the tunnel. Please find additional PMDD resources at the end of this book.

Premenstrual Syndrome (PMS)

In Chapter 7, we learned that there are over 150 symptoms of PMS. In this section, we'll focus on the mood-based premenstrual symptoms. While it's easy to simply pin the mood changes we may experience on our hormones, it is true that in the week or so before our periods begin, the cyclical decline in oestrogen, progesterone, serotonin and dopamine can have a negative effect on mood.[18] Decreased oestrogen levels result in the hypothalamus, one of the hormone control centres in our brain, releasing noradrenaline, one of our stress hormones which then triggers a decline in acetylcholine, dopamine and serotonin.[19] As our levels of progesterone decrease, so do our levels of GABA.

Here's a quick refresher on these neurotransmitters:

- **Acetylcholine:** a brain neurotransmitter with many functions, including supporting mental processes such as memory, learning, attention, motivation and cognition[20]
- **Dopamine:** a brain neurotransmitter that plays a role in behaviours involving motivation, punishment and reward, as well as cognitive functions involving attention, learning and memory and mood regulation[21]

- **Serotonin:** a neurotransmitter and a hormone, depending on where in the body it is used; most of our serotonin is found in our gut, where it helps to control digestion and bowel movements, and in the brain, where it regulates almost all our behavioural processes, including mood and sleep[22]
- **Gamma Aminobutyric Acid (GABA):** the primary inhibitory brain neurotransmitter, which decreases activity in our nervous system and has a calming effect[23]

In the late luteal phase of your menstrual cycle, you may start to experience mood swings, anxiety and depression, which can all manifest differently. You may experience all three. Let's talk about each of these and what you can do to support yourself if you feel like this.

Premenstrual Mood Swings

For some of us, the premenstrual drop in hormones and neurotransmitters can make us feel like we're off-kilter. Those of us that are normally quite even-keeled can find that our moods change rapidly. One moment you can feel fine, the next you can find yourself feeling more irritated than you usually would. Or you might find anger or rage bubbling closer to the surface and perhaps boiling over more easily. It could be that tears are more frequent.

It's important that we avoid pathologizing normal emotions and moods. Allow yourself to feel what you feel. If you feel that the anger, irritation or sadness is disproportionate to the situation, I encourage you to investigate this further.

Sorcha's Story

Sorcha came to see me because she didn't like who she became in the week before her period. She would find herself shouting at her husband over something she would have shrugged off the week before. She found herself becoming hypervigilant over her young son, keeping a beady eye on his every movement, when ordinarily she had a much more laissez-faire parenting style. By the time her period arrived, Sorcha's nerves were completely frayed.

Remember the veil of accommodation we talked about earlier in this chapter? I asked Sorcha to consider if she was having normal reactions to external situations. She pondered this and still felt that her reactions were disproportionate, so we began to investigate the cause of the premenstrual mood swings.

Sorcha told me that she would go to bed at 1am every night. After a day working and looking after her young child, she needed some time to herself, even if it was just an hour or two watching some bad television. We talked about the psychological phenomenon revenge bedtime procrastination,[24] where the individual goes to bed much later than intended in order to reclaim time and engage in the more pleasurable activities they hadn't been able to do during the day.[25] With this in mind, Sorcha started going to bed when she felt tired, which was usually around 10.30 or 11pm. She also started to approach her day differently, looking at it as less of a slog that she needed to push through and more as an opportunity to find moments of pleasure where she could.

I asked Sorcha to add more protein to her meals and increase the amount of fibre she ate each day, to give her gut some love and a bit of a helping hand in making serotonin. This also had the additional benefit of increasing the frequency of her bowel movements, as she had only been going every other day, if that. We then looked at how we could support ovulation so that Sorcha was producing enough progesterone to keep her post-ovulation oestrogen levels balanced. Getting more high-quality sleep was a big part of this. We also increased her vitamin D levels and added more vitamin E foods like spinach, pumpkin and sunflower seeds.

Slowly but surely, Sorcha noticed a decrease in the premenstrual rage and anxiety and had a better understanding of what she could do if this became an issue in the future.

Premenstrual Anxiety

In my work with clients, I see a spectrum when it comes to premenstrual anxiety. For some, it can look like avoidance of social situations and anything unfamiliar. For others, premenstrual anxiety can manifest more as self-doubt and criticism. You might find yourself worrying more, feeling more on edge, or second-guessing everything you do. You might find that if you already experience anxiety, your symptoms are heightened leading up to your period. This is called premenstrual exacerbation (PME), where the symptoms of an existing condition are worsened in the late luteal phase.

Some common symptoms of premenstrual anxiety include:

- Increased or uncontrollable worry
- Trouble relaxing / restlessness
- Feeling fearful
- Avoiding situations or people you would normally feel comfortable with
- Trouble sleeping
- Appetite changes
- Anxiety or panic attacks

If you relate to any of this, the first step is to recognize and acknowledge how you feel. Then start to notice when in your cycle the anxiety starts. Do you have any specific triggers? Does the anxiety decrease or cease when your period starts?

Our hormones and neurotransmitters are powerful, and it's normal to feel the effects of their decline in the late luteal phase. But there is a difference between feeling a little more self-critical and uncontrollable worry. If you find that premenstrual anxiety symptoms you're experiencing are becoming interruptive to your daily life, please speak to your doctor. Later in the chapter, we'll talk about how nutrition and lifestyle changes can support and reduce premenstrual anxiety symptoms.

Premenstrual Depression

Premenstrual depression feels different to premenstrual anxiety. In the seven to ten days before your period, you might find yourself sleeping more, more prone to tears, a little more forgetful or feeling apathetic about events and activities that would ordinarily excite you. As with premenstrual anxiety, we need to consider whether the premenstrual depression is an exacerbation (PME) of depression you already experience.

Some common symptoms of premenstrual depression include:

- Tearfulness
- Very low moods
- Appetite changes
- Forgetfulness
- Concentration issues
- Lack of energy / fatigue (remember, it's normal to have less energy before your period – here, we're looking at if you're really struggling to find the energy to do what you need to do)
- Apathy / lack of interest in activities and events that would normally excite you

If you feel like this before your period, it could be a sign from your body to slow down a little during the rest of your cycle. Energy depletion can manifest as the symptoms of premenstrual depression. Please speak to your doctor if you've been tracking your symptoms over two to three cycles, they don't shift a few days into your period and they are worsening.

Supporting Premenstrual Mood Changes Through Food and Lifestyle

What we eat each day, how much we sleep and how we move our bodies can help reduce the severity of the premenstrual drop in hormones and neurotransmitters. If we go into our late luteal phase having ovulated, made enough progesterone and we're giving our gut enough love each day, it can make the mood changes less severe. Regular physical movement, such as yoga, walking, Pilates, cycling and swimming are really helpful for enhancing mood, decreasing stress and increasing peace of mind.[26]

Give Your Gut Some Love

Throughout this book, we've talked about the importance of gut health for keeping oestrogen and progesterone in balance and for making enough serotonin, our happy hormone / neurotransmitter.

Here are seven ways to check if you're giving your gut enough love.

1. Do you find ways to include vegetables in most meals?
2. Are you eating enough high-protein foods like eggs, high-quality red meat, beans and pulses, cheese and fermented tofu, along with complex carbohydrates like sweet potato, rice and grains?
3. Are you eating enough vitamin B6 foods like banana, spinach, carrot, eggs and almonds?
4. Have you explored the world of nuts and seeds, in their different forms?
5. Do you know the difference between soluble and insoluble fibre?

6. Do you have a favourite fermented food or drink?
7. Are you giving your body the opportunity to absorb and digest your food well?
8. Are you taking breaks in between meals to let your motor migrating complex (MMC) do its thing?
9. Are you having a daily bowel movement, ideally in the morning?

As a nutritionist, I like to start with nutritional supports for premenstrual mood changes, but these may not always be enough or work as quickly as the client needs. Research has shown that gut bacteria produce the neurotransmitters that affect our mood during the late luteal phase: serotonin, dopamine, GABA and noradrenaline.[27] You might also like to add in a probiotic supplement with specific bacterial strains that research shows supports their positive effects on stress, anxiety and low mood. These include:

- Bifidobacterium longum 1714[28]
- Lactobacillus acidophilus Rosell-52[29]
- Bifidobacterium longum Rosell-175[30]
- Lactobacillus casei Shirota[31]
- Lactobacillus rhamnosus[32]

In the UK, you can find these strains in practitioner-grade probiotics from companies such as Bio-Kult, Optibac, Designs for Health, Nutri Advanced and BioCare. I recommend cycling between brands, taking them for three months at a time and leaving a one-month gap between them, as this introduces a variety of strains into your gut.

Sip on Some Green Tea (or a Matcha!)

L-theanine, an amino acid found in green tea and matcha (a powdered and more potent form of green tea) is a helpful way to increase concentration and find a sense of calmness. A small German study found that l-theanine supplementation was helpful for reducing anxiety and depression symptoms, as well as sleep problems. This study also found l-theanine beneficial for increasing cognitive function and verbal fluency.[33] In this study, the participants took 200mg a day for four weeks.

For my clients that supplement with l-theanine, I typically recommend 250mg a day, taken in the morning, for four weeks at a time, with a four-week break in between.

If you want to add matcha or green tea, remember they contain caffeine. Although we metabolize the caffeine in matcha and green tea differently to that in coffee, if you are sensitive to caffeine, limit your intake to the morning.

All of the Lights

Earlier in this chapter, we talked about the circadian rhythm and the benefits of exposing your eyes to bright lights first thing in the morning. This also improves feelings of alertness and vitality, as well as helping to increase serotonin levels.

In the summer months, get outdoors as early as you can, even if it's just popping your head outside for a few minutes. The light exposure to the retina in your eyes and on your skin triggers the release of serotonin.[34] How cool is that?

If it's not easy to get outside in the winter months, it may be worth investing in a light therapy box or a SAD lamp to boost serotonin levels.[35] Make sure the lamp has at least 10,000 lux or lumens, so the light source is intense enough to mimic real sunlight. And don't forget to open your curtains wide and let the light in!

TRY THE 4–7–8 BREATHING TECHNIQUE

Dr Andrew Weil, the renowned integrative medicine doctor, developed the 4–7–8 breathing technique[36] as a way of shifting our nervous system and reducing stress and anxiety. If you'd like to try it, follow the steps below.

1. Find a comfortable, relaxing place to lie or sit.
2. Place the tip of your tongue against the ridge of tissue just behind your upper front teeth and keep it there for the entire exercise. Keep your tongue in place throughout the practice. You might find it easier to purse your lips.
3. Let your lips part and exhale completely through your mouth, making a whoosh sound.
4. Close your mouth and inhale quietly through your nose for 4 counts.
5. Hold your breath for 7 counts.
6. Exhale completely through your mouth, making a whoosh sound for 8 counts.
7. Start a new 4–7–8 cycle of breath.

Remember that like period pain, premenstrual mood changes, anxiety and depression may be common, but they're not normal. This may be the first time you've ever heard anything like this. Begin to take note of how you feel after you ovulate, jotting down any major mood changes. When you experience these, ask yourself whether it's a normal reaction or if these changes might be heightened by shifting hormones during the second half of your menstrual cycle. You might find it helpful to take notes. After a few months, you'll start to see patterns to your mood changes, which should hopefully help you better understand what you're experiencing, so that you can get the help you need.

CHAPTER 10

Where Has My Period Gone? – What to Do About Missing Periods

When the timing and regularity of your period changes, it can be very disconcerting, can't it? Picture this: your period usually comes like clockwork every 30 days. You can plan your life around it and you do. You knew when to schedule your wedding and honeymoon, when to schedule your last three appraisals and even when to schedule date night! In the last six months, your period has been all over the place. You had a 45-day cycle, then a 60-day cycle and your last cycle was 90 days! You find it unnerving because your period was always a certainty, and now it's not. You're worried it's going to disappear altogether. Far from being a curse, you would welcome the return of your period.

Do you relate to this at all?

We've talked about painful periods and heavy periods – now let's talk about irregular and missing periods. We know that periods and menstrual cycles are one of our five vital signs and when our period is irregular or missing, we need to investigate.

In this chapter, we'll talk about the reasons for an irregular or missing period: PCOS and functional hypothalamic amenorrhea. And remember, thyroid issues such as hypo-

and hyperthyroidism can lead to irregular and missing periods, so if this is something you're struggling with, I urge you to get your thyroid tested. Flip back to Chapter 3 for more information about this.

PCOS

Polycystic ovarian syndrome, or PCOS for short, is one of the most common women's reproductive health conditions, affecting up to 10 per cent of women of reproductive age in the UK.[1] If not treated, the symptoms of PCOS can lead to complications including difficulty conceiving due to irregular menstrual cycles and lack of ovulation, increased risk for type 2 diabetes and cardiovascular issues.[2]

PCOS can be tricky to diagnose because it has been defined as a syndrome. This means that there is a collection of different symptoms (we also see this with PMS!), and no single symptom is sufficient for clinical diagnosis. Because PCOS is a syndrome with a variety of symptoms, it's essential not to rely on ultrasound results as the single diagnostic tool. If an ultrasound has been the basis of your PCOS diagnosis, I encourage you to ask your doctor to investigate further with appropriate blood tests. I've outlined the tests you may consider asking for later in this chapter.

Remember that ovarian cysts don't always equal PCOS. It is possible to have PCOS without the presence of ovarian cysts and, conversely, to have ovarian cysts and not have PCOS. Sounds tricky, doesn't it? Not to worry, you'll feel a lot clearer once you get to the end of this chapter.

Symptoms of PCOS typically begin to appear around puberty. Some of the most common symptoms are:[3]

- Hirsutism, or excess hair growth on the chest, abdomen, back and face, which is typically dark and coarse
- Acne on the chest, chin, jawline and / or back
- Oily skin

- Hair thinning or male pattern baldness
- Highly irregular periods with long menstrual cycles (typically 35+ days)
- Menstrual cycles with no ovulation
- Blood sugar dysregulation and strong sugar cravings
- High cholesterol levels
- Weight gain and difficulty losing weight
- Depression and / or anxiety
- Difficulty conceiving due to long menstrual cycles and irregular periods

Because there is such a wide range of symptoms, PCOS can look drastically different from person to person, which is why there is truly no one-size-fits-all when it comes to treatment and symptom management. As we'll discuss later in this chapter, there are four major types of PCOS, each with predominant symptoms, which may overlap. Understanding your PCOS type will help you get the most appropriate treatment that addresses the root cause and the dominant symptoms first.

The exact cause of PCOS is not currently known, but family history is a key consideration, as the likelihood of diagnosis is increased in those with a first-degree female family member with the syndrome. Some researchers suggest that environmental factors have a role in the development of PCOS,[4] hypothesizing that BPA and other androgen-disrupting chemicals may accumulate to a greater extent in individuals with PCOS because of decreased hormone metabolism in the liver. This would exacerbate symptoms of excessive androgen production and insulin resistance.

PCOS is typically a diagnosis of exclusion. If you suspect you have it, your doctor or healthcare practitioner will look for two out of the following three symptoms as a way of diagnosing you, using a diagnostic tool called the Rotterdam Criteria:[5]

1. Irregular periods
2. Excess androgen levels (androgens refer to testosterone, DHEAS and androstenedione)
3. Polycystic ovaries on pelvic ultrasound, with at least one ovary having 12 or more follicles of 2–9mm in diameter and / or ovarian volume of greater than 10ml

This method of diagnosis has come up against some controversy. Some say that it lumps all the PCOS phenotypes together, as many PCOS patients do not have an androgen excess, and instead have high insulin levels.[6] Many of those with PCOS do not have polycystic ovaries on ultrasound, and yet they still have this condition because they have the other symptoms of PCOS, including long menstrual cycles / irregular periods and high androgen levels or high insulin levels on testing.

Conversely, polycystic ovaries (PCO) occur in 20 to 30 per cent of women,[7] but these women do not always have PCOS. This means that a PCOS diagnosis cannot be made from an ultrasound indicating PCO alone.

The wide variety in PCOS phenotypes[8] means that there's no standard go-to treatment. It's helpful to know the type of PCOS you have, so you can get the appropriate treatment that starts by addressing the key symptoms you're experiencing within the specific PCOS type. Knowing your type can help ensure that you are correctly diagnosed. Some of the key symptoms of PCOS are also symptoms of other conditions. For example, other causes of anovulation, or lack of ovulation, include:[9]

- Hyperprolactinemia, or high prolactin levels[10]
- Hypothyroidism, an underactive thyroid
- Congenital adrenal hyperplasia (CAH)
- Pituitary gland failure
- Hypothalamic amenorrhea (HA), which we'll discuss later in this chapter

- High levels of sustained physical and emotional stress, which we covered in Chapter 6, as this can impact our ability to ovulate each menstrual cycle
- Perimenopause and menopause

Other causes of high androgen levels include:

- Congenital adrenal hyperplasia (CAH)
- High prolactin
- An imbalance of androgen hormones
- Menopause
- Cushing's disease
- Adrenal tumours
- Ovarian tumours

Other causes of high insulin levels / insulin resistance include:

- A waistline over 88cm (35in)
- Gestational diabetes
- Nonalcoholic fatty liver disease
- Type 2 diabetes
- Acromegaly
- Some medications, including steroids, antipsychotics and HIV medications

To ensure that you are being treated for the right PCOS type, you want to make sure you have a wide range of blood tests, including the following:

Blood Test Category	Blood Marker
Blood sugar	Fasting insulin
	HbA1c
	Fasting glucose
Cholesterol	Total cholesterol
	LDL
	HDL
	Triglycerides
Androgens	Serum free testosterone
	Serum total testosterone
	Serum androstenedione
	Serum DHEAS
Other sex hormones	Serum oestrogen, luteinizing hormone (LH) and follicle stimulating hormone (FSH) on day 2 or 3 of the menstrual cycle
	Serum progesterone and oestrogen 7 days after ovulation
	Serum SHBG
	Serum prolactin
Inflammation	CRP
Thyroid	TSH
	Free T4
	Free T3
	Reverse T3
	TPO
	TgAB

Note: if your cycles are very long or irregular, you can have your oestrogen, progesterone, LH and FSH levels tested irrespective of cycle day. Your doctor or healthcare practitioner will be looking for variations from expected optimal ranges, including an elevated LH to FSH ratio. This also helps to rule out hypothalamic amenorrhea (HA), perimenopause and premature ovarian failure.

PCOS can have an impact on fertility, because high insulin levels from insulin resistance, hyperandrogenism and altered ovarian hormone signalling can disrupt follicle growth into a mature egg.[11] This can then lead to irregular menstrual cycles, anovulation and the accumulation of small antral follicles, or partially developed follicles, around the edge of the ovary. It must be said that there are women with PCOS who go on to have healthy pregnancies and childbirth, so if you have been diagnosed with PCOS, please don't automatically expect that you will struggle with infertility.

Nutrition and Lifestyle Foundations for All PCOS Types

Here are some nutrition and lifestyle foundations that can support PCOS symptoms. These changes can apply to everyone, as well as specific advice for the different types.

Balance Your Blood Sugar Levels

Meals that balance blood sugar, detailed in the later section, provide a healthy foundation for any type of PCOS.

What we eat, the quality of our sleep and how we move our bodies have a significant impact on our blood sugar levels. Many with PCOS can feel as though they're going on a rollercoaster throughout the day, using sugar and caffeine to prop up their energy levels and mood. As we discussed in Chapter 3, meals that include a combination of high-quality protein, fats, fibres and greens help us feel fuller for longer and stop us going up and down this blood sugar rollercoaster.

This would mean moving away from a bowl of cereal and milk for breakfast and having a bowl of porridge / oatmeal with berries and a tablespoon of nut butter or a slice of a frittata that's been made with lots of greens, some cheese and smoked salmon.

When we eat in a way that balances our blood sugar levels after each meal, they stop going up and down dramatically and instead resemble a valley of rolling hills, gently rising and falling.

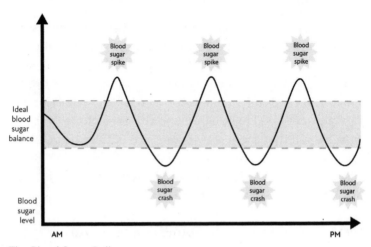

The Blood Sugar Rollercoaster

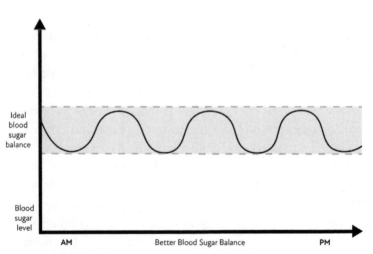

Blood Sugar Balance

Be Mindful of the Impact of Stress

Many of my clients are surprised at what a negative effect stress can have on our health. So often, we race through action-packed days without a chance to catch our breath. We're often more stressed than we realize. Imagine a staircase: as our stress levels increase, our nervous systems work harder and harder to manage the effects of higher cortisol levels on our health. As we move higher and higher up the stress staircase, the harder our nervous systems work to bring us back to homeostasis, or the status quo, and our body adapts to this new normal. For a recap of the different types of stress, go back to Chapter 3.

As we'll learn later in this chapter, high cortisol levels negatively impact three types of PCOS: high androgen, insulin-resistant and inflammatory PCOS. High cortisol can lead to high androgen levels, high insulin levels and increased inflammation, exacerbating the symptoms of each of these types of PCOS.

I want you to be honest about how stressed you really are, the sources of your stress and what you can realistically do to reduce it. Many of my clients look at stress reduction as yet another task on their to-do list. I ask them to think differently, instead looking at what they can sprinkle throughout their day: five to ten minutes outside first thing in the morning; deep, calming breaths regularly during the day; standing up and shaking out their arms and legs vigorously to shift the nervous system; a screen-free lunch eaten seated at the table. Start with one thing and do it regularly for a few weeks. Notice how you feel. If it helps, keep going. If it doesn't, try something different.

MOVE YOUR BODY DIFFERENTLY OVER THE COURSE OF A WEEK

Think about the way you exercise or move your body. How much variety is there in your exercise routine? If you've got into a rut, you're not alone. As we'll learn later in this chapter, too much high-impact exercise, including running, spinning and HIIT, can increase cortisol levels. We feel great after we're done because of the release of endorphins, but the stress of this type of exercise on the body also increases cortisol levels. In the last section, we learned about the impact of cortisol on PCOS: too much, too often is not helpful.

Could you mix things up a little, adding in brisk walking for at least 20 minutes, five days a week and resistance training at least three days a week? This variety will reduce cortisol release from exercise, making way for the health benefits, including better insulin sensitivity, reduced inflammation and lower androgen levels.

High Androgen or Adrenal PCOS

This is the first of the four types of PCOS we'll be looking at. You may see this type of PCOS called high androgen PCOS in some places or adrenal PCOS in others. High cortisol levels, which are produced in the adrenals (those tiny little glands that sit on top of the kidneys), cause androgen levels to increase. A vicious cycle can persist with this type of PCOS:

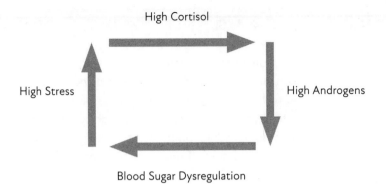

High Cortisol

High Stress

High Androgens

Blood Sugar Dysregulation

Stress, Cortisol and Androgens: A Vicious Cycle

Those with this type of PCOS typically have some of the classic PCOS signs and symptoms: cystic acne along the jawline, cheeks, back and / or chest; dark, coarse hair along the jawline, chest and abdomen; oily skin; and hair loss, including male pattern baldness. If you have this type of PCOS, you might find that you also have some of the other symptoms associated with the other PCOS types, but the high androgen symptoms predominate.

When you get your blood tested, you will see high serum androgen levels. According to research, circulating total and free testosterone as well as DHEAS levels are elevated in 50 to 75 per cent of women with PCOS.[12] High androgens can be caused by insulin resistance and high insulin levels, because they cause a reduction in sex hormone-binding globulin (SHBG) levels, which then lead to an increase in androgen levels.[13] In other words, we see another vicious cycle between insulin resistance and high androgen levels, which then has a negative effect on ovulation and the ability to have regular menstrual cycles.

Nutrition and Lifestyle Support for High Androgen PCOS

Trial Removing Dairy for a Short Time
It's become a bit of a truism in the PCOS world that removing dairy will heal some of the symptoms. As with everything in this book, it's essential to consider your own bio-individuality. Some will respond well to taking out cow's milk dairy for a short amount of time, and with others, it will have zero impact. Cow's milk dairy contains a compound called insulin growth factor (IGF-1) which can increase sebum, leading to oily skin and increased acne.[14] A month-long trial can help to normalize skin and reduce acne. The key word here is trial. Dairy is very nutrient-rich and can be a great addition to our daily meals. In my clinical practice, my clients also work on their gut health, which can often be compromised in PCOS. By improving gut health and nutrient absorption, it is easier to slowly add dairy back in after a month-long exclusion. If you have a history of disordered eating or a previous eating disorder, I suggest using the other high androgen PCOS nutrition supports first.

Eat Foods with DIM
Diindolylmethane (DIM) is a phytonutrient found mainly in cruciferous vegetables[15] such as broccoli, pak choi/bok choy, cauliflower, cabbage, greens, kale, Brussels sprouts and kohlrabi. This phytonutrient is beneficial for this type of PCOS because it acts as an antiandrogen,[16] helping to reduce testosterone levels.

Eat at least two to three servings of these vegetables a day for at least three months. If you're not sure what a serving looks like, flip back to Chapter 5 for examples.

Drink Spearmint Tea
A small Turkish research study found that spearmint tea has antiandrogenic properties,[17] which means it can help reduce free and total testosterone levels. This can lead to

a reduction in the coarse, dark facial and body hair that characterizes this type of PCOS.

Try drinking two cups of spearmint tea each day. For each cup, you can use 2 tsp of fresh spearmint leaves in a cup of boiling water. Let it steep for ten minutes, strain and drink.

Drink Green Tea or Matcha

I can't say enough about matcha. It has so many benefits, including its antiandrogenic properties. Green tea contains an antioxidant called epigallocatechin gallate (EGCG), which inhibits the conversion of testosterone into a more toxic form called DHT (5-alpha dihydrotestosterone) by reducing the amount of 5-alpha reductase, the enzyme that drives this conversion.[18]

Matcha, which is powdered green tea, is more potent than green tea, so you may choose to drink this for more EGCG. Be mindful that matcha does contain more caffeine, so avoid drinking it late in the day. Try swapping your morning coffee, which can increase cortisol levels, for a matcha latte instead.

Address Stress Levels

We know that high stress levels can exacerbate the symptoms of adrenal / high androgen PCOS, so it's important to take an honest look at the stress you're experiencing and put active measures in place to address them.

Yoga, mindfulness, walking and a more intentional way of working can be beneficial in reducing stress levels. Deep breathing is another important tool that can be used during moments of stress.

Try sitting down with your feet flat on the ground. Place your hands on your lap or your chest. Take four counts of breath in through your nose and then four counts of breath out through your nose. Do this as many times as you need.

Pump Some Iron

A 2016 Brazilian study asked 45 women with PCOS to perform progressive resistance training (PRT) three times a week for four months. When the study ended, these women had reduced testosterone and fasting glucose levels.[19] Resistance training doesn't necessarily mean lifting heavy weights (although that's fun too!). You could use the exercise machines in the gym, exercise bands, kettlebells or even your own bodyweight. Find something that suits you and incorporate some form of resistance training into your movement schedule for at least 20 minutes, three times a week.

Supplements

Zinc has been shown to inhibit androgen receptors, as well as helping to properly metabolize androgens away from DHT, a more toxic form of testosterone that contributes to male pattern baldness and acne.[20]

Additionally, zinc is also beneficial for ovarian function, which, when improved, decreases androgen levels. It also supports healthy progesterone production, which then acts as a natural androgen blocker.

A good multivitamin will have at least 15mg, and a healthcare practitioner can advise if there is any benefit from additional zinc supplementation. You can also increase the amount of zinc in your meals with foods like high-quality beef and lamb, oysters and other seafood, and pumpkin seeds.

Insulin-resistant PCOS

Insulin resistance is a common feature of the majority of the four PCOS types. It's a term you've probably heard a lot, but potentially aren't sure exactly what it means. In a nutshell, insulin resistance means that the cells in the muscles, fat and liver don't respond well to receiving insulin produced in the pancreas. This means that these cells are unable to use glucose from the blood for energy. This creates a pattern where the pancreas then makes more insulin to help move glucose into the blood and the cells continue to resist this insulin, leaving the sugar in the blood and persistently high insulin levels. Eventually, the cells start to ignore these signals and the pancreas can't produce as much insulin, which then increases the risk for type 2 diabetes.

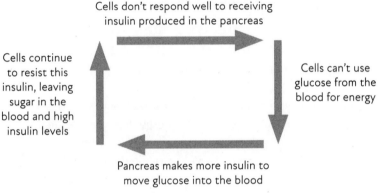

Cells don't respond well to receiving insulin produced in the pancreas

Cells continue to resist this insulin, leaving sugar in the blood and high insulin levels

Cells can't use glucose from the blood for energy

Pancreas makes more insulin to move glucose into the blood

Insulin Resistance

In PCOS, high insulin levels and insulin resistance is noted in 50 to 70 per cent of patients[21] and can cause or exacerbate high androgen levels and vice versa. The high insulin levels both cause the theca cells in the ovary to produce androgens and can increase the number of theca cells, which means that the ovary can produce more androgens. This will then affect ovulation, which leads to anovulatory (lack of ovulation) or irregular menstrual cycles. In this PCOS type, insulin resistance and its symptoms tend to dominate over the symptoms of the other PCOS phenotypes.

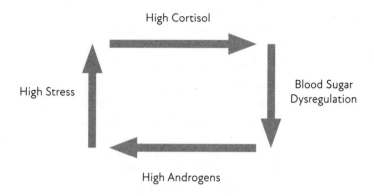

High Cortisol

High Stress

Blood Sugar
Dysregulation

High Androgens

Cortisol, Blood Sugar Dysregulation and Androgens

With this type of PCOS, you might notice that you crave sweets or that you have sudden energy dips that require a snack to get you going again. In extreme cases, you might feel dizzy and faint if you don't eat regularly.

Nutrition and Lifestyle Support for Insulin-resistant PCOS

Support Blood Sugar Balance
With insulin-resistant PCOS, it is essential to reduce the pressure on the pancreas and the amount of insulin it is required to produce. Simple dietary changes can be highly effective in increasing insulin sensitivity. One way of doing this is eating three meals a day that are nutritionally dense, with a balance between high-quality protein, fibre, greens and healthy fats. This helps support blood sugar balance and decreases the number of blood sugar spikes and drops that lead to sugar cravings. The Balanced Plate that we talked about in Chapter 3 and earlier in this chapter will form the foundation of eating to reduce insulin resistance, making sure that each meal has enough to satiate you and help increase insulin sensitivity.

In the PCOS world, one-size-fits-all thinking can persist, especially around carbohydrates. You don't have to exclude carbohydrates to reduce insulin resistance. And remember, we need carbohydrates for many bodily functions, including for a healthy thyroid. When we include enough high-quality fat and protein in our meals, we can support our body in becoming more sensitive to insulin.

A great way to implement this is to start by looking at what you include in each of your daily meals.

A typical lunch and dinner plate could be:

- ¼ high-quality protein (e.g. 80g / 3oz free-range, organic beef, lamb or poultry, lentils, chickpeas/garbanzo beans or quinoa)
- ½ green leafy vegetables (e.g. 70g / 2½oz spinach, 30g / 1oz kale, 90g / 3oz steamed broccoli or 120g / 4oz carrots)
- ¼ complex carbohydrate with lots of fibre (e.g. sweet potato, carrots, parsnips, brown rice)
- A small portion of good fats, such as 1 tbsp almond butter, ½ avocado, 1 tbsp olive oil

A typical breakfast could be:

- A 2- or 3-egg omelette with a handful of greens, grated carrot and grated cheese, cooked in butter or olive oil
- A smoothie made with almond milk, a handful of greens, 1 tbsp almond butter, a handful of berries, 1 tbsp pumpkin or chia seeds, 1 scoop of hemp protein powder

Increase Fibre to Support Blood Sugar Balance
Studies have shown dietary fibres has a positive effect on managing blood sugar levels.[22] Ideally, we want to be eating at least 30g of fibre every day. What does this mean in practice?

- Include two types of vegetable in every meal, emphasizing green vegetables, if possible

- Avoid peeling vegetables such as potatoes, carrots, parsnips and sweet potatoes, as the skin contains a lot of valuable fibre
- Eat a variety of fibre sources, including legumes, fruit, vegetables, brown rice, brown bread and brown pasta
- Add nuts and seeds to your meals, including flaxseed, which has been found to reduce insulin levels[23]

Move Your Body

At least 150 minutes of either resistance or endurance physical activity a week[24] (which is just over 20 minutes a day), alongside a modified way of eating that includes the changes I talked about in the last section, can reduce high insulin levels and increase insulin sensitivity. Please bear in mind that the type of exercise does matter. I'm always keen for my clients with both insulin-resistant and high androgen PCOS to move their bodies in different ways rather than over-relying on HIIT and other high-impact exercise as their only form of exercise. Research shows that HIIT can be beneficial for reducing insulin resistance in PCOS,[25] but we need to bear in mind that it can increase cortisol and subsequently insulin levels. It's better to do a mix of exercise including resistance training each week.[26] And don't forget low-impact exercise like swimming, walking, yoga and Pilates for their positive effects on our nervous systems, which then helps to reduce cortisol levels.

Create a Calm Eating Environment

What we eat is important, but how we eat is too. The next time you eat, notice how quickly you chew your food, the eating environment (are you eating in front of the TV or eating standing up?) and how you feel when you finish your food. Eating too quickly and in a rushed way can increase cortisol and can have a negative effect on blood sugar levels, as well as quality of digestion.

The next time you eat, spend time creating the calmest possible environment. Chew each bite of food between five and ten times, put your fork and knife down between bites and look at your meal as an opportunity to take time for yourself, rather than rushing through to the next thing on your to-do list.

Supplements

In conventional medicine, metformin is typically used with insulin-resistant PCOS to support improved glucose tolerance and increase insulin sensitivity. Some women can experience side effects from this medication, including diarrhoea, abdominal discomfort and sleepiness.

Research shows that myo-inositol combined with folate can be just as effective as metformin. A 2016 Turkish study found that fasting glucose, LDL, DHEAS, total cholesterol and prolactin levels decreased significantly[27] with myo-inositol and folic acid supplementation. Additionally, there was also a significant drop in anti-Mullerian hormone (AMH) levels, ovarian volume, ovarian antral follicle and total antral follicle counts, which have positive effects on restoring healthy ovulation and regulating menstrual cycles.

If you are considering this route, please work with a practitioner who can recommend the right dosage levels. If in doubt, choose a supplement with folate rather than folic acid (the synthetic version of folate).

Inflammatory PCOS

This third type of PCOS is primarily driven by chronic inflammation. As we've talked about throughout this book, inflammation is typically something that we want to happen. When it is acute, or short-term, it helps us heal cuts and wounds and helps our immune system fight bacteria and viruses. When we are chronically inflamed, it means that our immune system continues to act as though there is a threat, which then starts to damage cells in our bodies.

With inflammatory PCOS, we see that chronic low-grade levels of inflammation can increase androgen levels and have a negative effect on ovulation.[28] In this type of PCOS, there isn't the insulin resistance that is present with high androgen and insulin-resistant PCOS, so treatment options will focus on reducing the inflammation that is causing hormone disruption.

You will typically see high CRP levels on a blood test result, alongside high levels of the various androgen (testosterone, androstenedione and DHEAS) markers we would be exploring with high androgen PCOS.

Nutrition and Lifestyle Support for Inflammatory PCOS

Add Anti-Inflammatory Foods
Food is a valuable way of reducing the body's inflammatory response and can help bring down the inflammatory markers that can, in turn, increase androgen levels. For more detail about the variety of anti-inflammatory foods you can add into your meals, turn to Chapter 8.

Try adding these foods to every meal of the day to continually give your body anti-inflammatory support.

Eat the Rainbow
As we've discussed earlier in this book, eating a rainbow of fruits and vegetables every day will add valuable antioxidants that help our bodies reduce chronic inflammation.[29]

Give yourself the challenge of adding in a new-to-you fruit or vegetable every week and making your plate as brightly coloured as possible.

Prioritize Getting Your 40 Winks
How did you feel when you woke up this morning? Rested or like you could fall back into bed and sleep for another few hours? So many of us get into a cycle of skimping on sleep in the week, running on empty and using caffeine and sugar

to prop up our energy levels during the day. Then we resolve to catch up on sleep at the weekend. This pattern creates a sleep deficit that has a negative effect on our health, especially with inflammatory PCOS.

Sleep is the foundation of our health. When we're deprived of it (sleep deprivation is classified as getting fewer than six hours of sleep a night), it can increase inflammation and raise cortisol levels. Research shows that acute sleep loss can increase inflammatory markers,[30] which can then exacerbate the symptoms of this form of PCOS.

Getting better sleep is one of the best things you can do for your health. Did you know that great sleep starts at the beginning of the day with exposure to daylight? This sends signals to our brain to say it's time to reduce the high cortisol levels that helped wake us up.[31] Exposure to daylight also helps set our circadian rhythm (our body clock), so that our brain knows that it's daytime and it's time to be awake. When the evening comes, the darkness signals to our brains that it's time to start making melatonin, the hormone that helps us get to sleep and stay asleep. Unfortunately, bright lights and blue light from laptops, phones, tablets and televisions can reduce the amount of melatonin our brain makes.[32]

And then we add busyness until the end of the day, giving us a recipe for restless, poor-quality sleep. Think about what you do in the evening. Is it a race to fit everything you want to do into the day? Are you busy right until bedtime? We need to give our brain and body the opportunity to unwind at the end of the day. Mental busyness means that our brains don't get any downtime and we can end up tossing and turning and sleeping badly.

Fortunately, there's a lot you can do.

1. Make your bedroom as inviting as possible so that when you go to bed you feel relaxed and comfortable. One small thing you can do each morning is to make your

bed. Imagine walking into your bedroom at night seeing a made bed waiting for you to climb into it. Sounds lovely, doesn't it?

2. Create a digital sunset by shutting down all your blue-light-producing devices around 30 to 60 minutes before you go to bed. If that seems too hard, you could also get a pair of blue-light-blocking glasses that you wear when you're watching TV or using your computer, tablet or phone at night.

3. Create a bedtime routine for yourself to help reduce your mental load at the end of the day. Our brain loves routine (did you know that about 40 to 45 per cent of what we do each day is based on routine?)[33] and the anticipation of what's to come at bedtime can help your brain start to unwind. Your bedtime routine doesn't need to be complicated. It could be washing your face, brushing your teeth, putting on pyjamas and reading a good book in bed. It could be putting some lavender sleep spray on your pillows for a deeper night's sleep. Or it could be some self-pleasure or sex with your partner – an orgasm is a lovely way to unwind before bed!

Address Stress Levels

As we learned in Chapter 2, physical and emotional stress activates the hypothalamic–pituitary–adrenal (HPA) axis and the sympathetic nervous system, raising our cortisol levels. Our bodies are always trying to find a way to come back into homeostasis, or balance.[34] When we are chronically and intensely stressed, our immune system becomes overactive, which then contributes to, and exacerbates, the chronic low-grade inflammation inherent in this type of PCOS.

If you haven't already, be honest about the stress you're experiencing and put active measures in place to address them.

As we discussed previously, yoga, mindfulness, walking and a more intentional way of working can be beneficial in reducing stress levels. Deep breathing is another important tool that can be used during moments of stress.

Try sitting down with your feet flat on the ground. Place your hands on your lap or your chest. Breath in deeply through your nose, then sigh it all out through your mouth.

Supplements

Glutathione is known as the master antioxidant. It works to reduce chronic inflammation and support our body's natural immune function.[35]

N-acetylcysteine (NAC) and alpha-lipoic acid (ALA)[36] both help increase the amount of glutathione our body produces, which then works to reduce chronic inflammation.

Work with a practitioner to understand the right dosages for you.

Post-Pill PCOS

This type of PCOS is the result of taking hormonal birth control. You may have found that your menstrual cycles and periods were normal and regular prior to going on the Pill and since you've been taking it or since coming off, you've started experiencing some of the PCOS symptoms we've talked about in this chapter.

When you take the Pill, it suppresses communication between the ovaries and the brain, which then stops ovulation. After coming off the Pill, this suppressed communication can persist, leading to a delay in the return of menstruation. Additionally, there can also be a rise in androgens after coming off some forms of the birth control pill. Finally, post-Pill PCOS may also be the result of undiagnosed PCOS prior to going on the Pill.

If this is what you think is happening for you, go back up to the high androgen section of this chapter and follow the recommendations there.

You will also want to make sure you're getting all the nutrients that are depleted by the Pill: the minerals zinc, magnesium and selenium, and vitamins B9 (folate), B6, B12, B2, C and E.[37] In Chapters 4 to 7, you will find tables that go through how to increase most of these vitamins and minerals through the food you eat. I also recommend taking a high-quality multivitamin to increase your body's stores of these nutrients. In the UK, Planet Organic, Revital and Whole Foods are great places to shop for a high-quality, practitioner-grade multivitamin.

Additionally, you will also want to look at supporting your gut health, as hormonal birth control can be disruptive to the health of the gut microbiome and the oestrogen metabolism that takes place there.[38] Flip to Chapter 8 for more information about how to support your gut health.

Graínne's Story

Graínne had always been sporty, playing team sports in elementary and high school, eventually going on to play football quite seriously in university. She trained hard, trying to balance her athletic endeavours with her schoolwork and a bit of social life. When Graínne's period arrived at 13, it was a monthly annoyance that she felt slowed her down and got in the way of how hard she could play on the pitch.

After a few years, Graínne noticed that her period had mysteriously disappeared. She saw this as a blessing in disguise because it meant she didn't need to adjust her training schedule anymore. She continued to train hard, adjusting her food intake to reduce carbohydrates, which she felt made her sluggish.

Graínne would have happily gone on with no period, but she started learning more about anatomy and physiology as part of her sports science degree. Although she was happy not to deal with what she saw as the blood and mess of having a period, she realized that missing out on the hormonal side of menstruation and the menstrual cycle would be having an impact on her performance on the pitch.

When we started working together, Gráinne had mixed feelings about trying to get her period back. Our work together focused on three areas: giving her body enough nutrients to support all the activity she was doing; changing her mindset around food, away from something she needed to burn off through exercise and toward something that could be pleasurable; and helping Gráinne find ways to support her body and brain so they felt safe enough to have a period and ovulate.

Gráinne was stuck in the mindset that carbohydrates were bad and would cause her to put on weight. I spent time educating her about the different types of carbohydrates and reorienting her thinking about what was on her plate, with a focus on protein, fat, fibre and greens. For at least three months, Gráinne had to actively remind herself to include foods like sweet potatoes, brown rice, carrots and couscous in her meals. She also discovered a new love for a range of fruits like mango, grapes and bananas that she had previously dismissed as too sugary.

We also made sure Gráinne was getting all the nutrients needed for a healthy menstrual cycle: iron, copper, vitamin A, magnesium, selenium, B6, C, zinc, iodine, B12, E and potassium, so that when her period did eventually come back, she would have a head start.

I was careful to manage Gráinne's expectations around when her period might return. It could take up to two years or longer, so Gráinne needed to be ready for this.

I also asked Gráinne to stop exercising above and beyond the training schedule required by her coaches, as often she would go on long runs on her days off, never really giving her body the opportunity to recover.

Gráinne and I spent three months working together working on all the foundations that would help her body feel safe enough to have a period and ovulate again. Six months later, I had a hopeful email from her saying, "Le'Nise, I've been following all of your recommendations to the letter and guess what? My period finally came back!"

Hypothalamic Amenorrhea (HA)

Our period is one of our vital signs, so when it goes missing, alarm bells should ring. If our periods stop and we're not on hormonal birth control, menopausal, pregnant or breastfeeding, we need to ask ourselves what could be happening that would prevent our bodies from feeling safe enough to menstruate. Not having a period has an impact on several of our body's systems, including the cardiovascular and skeletal, as well as our brain, thyroid, skin and reproductive organs. Hypothalamic amenorrhea (HA) is one of the most common causes of secondary amenorrhea, or missing periods, and occurs in 1–2 per cent of women of reproductive age.[39] The three most common causes of HA are:[40]

1. **Weight and food:** losing or gaining weight too quickly, ongoing restriction of nutrients and calories, under-eating and a current eating disorder or disordered eating
2. **Exercise:** over-exercising without giving the body enough recovery time
3. **Stress:** extended time of prolonged stress or trauma, a sudden shock or trauma

At the heart of this is the hypothalamus, one of the endocrine glands in the brain. Through what is called the HPO axis (hypothalamic–pituitary–ovarian), the hypothalamus signals via GnRH (gonadotropin-releasing hormone) to the pituitary gland, which then signals to the ovaries via FSH and LH that it's safe for the body to carry out the reproductive functions of ovulation and menstruation by making enough hormones like oestrogen and progesterone.[41] This affects our hunger hormones leptin and ghrelin. Leptin is the hormone that signals fullness and ghrelin is our hunger hormone. A 1998 study found that women with HA have lower levels of leptin after eating and higher levels of cortisol in general.[42] Prolonged high levels of cortisol can dysregulate hunger and satiety signals, perpetuating the cycle.

If your period is currently missing and you've ruled out PCOS (HA is sometimes misdiagnosed as PCOS because missing periods can be thought of as just very long menstrual cycles), then it's valuable to understand what could be causing this. To make sure you're getting the correct diagnosis, please make sure that your doctor or health practitioner runs a full range of blood tests.

If you have HA, you need to understand what could be causing your body to feel unsafe enough to stop menstruating.

- Are you eating enough? Eating too few carbohydrates or fats can cause our periods to go missing
- Are you over-exercising? This is one of the most common causes of missing periods in female athletes and is its own subcategory of HA called athletic amenorrhea[43]
- Are you stressed? Are you in a traumatic environment or is there unresolved trauma from your past?

Remember, you don't have to deal with this on your own. There is a mental aspect of HA that must be addressed for true healing to take place. If you believe your HA is the result of an eating disorder or disordered eating, I strongly recommend that you seek out professional help. The UK eating disorder charity BEAT[44] (or NEDA in the US[45]) are good starting places to learn how to ask for help and the type of treatment you should expect. If you believe your HA is the result of stress and / or trauma, I suggest finding a therapist who can support you. The British Association for Counselling and Psychotherapy[46] (or the American Counselling Association in the US[47]) is a good resource for finding a therapist in your local area or online.

In her 2016 book *No Period. Now What?*, the biologist Nicola J. Rinaldi says that "the fundamental goal is recovery of your health and fertility (and for many, to get pregnant). To get to that point, you need to supply yourself with energy not just for your current day-to-day needs, but also to replenish your body after months or years of underfueling."[48]

If you believe your HA is the result of overly restrictive eating, one part of HA recovery that can be challenging is becoming more open-minded to eating a wider variety of foods again. Many HA recovery experts advocate an approach that asks you to eat at least 2,500 calories a day. I believe that basing your recovery around a specific calorie target is problematic because it can lead you to another type of restrictive eating that focuses strictly on making sure you're eating enough calories. I would rather you move to a type of eating that focuses on eating enough of the foods that nourish you, helps you feel full and satisfied and helps your body feel safe enough to have a period and ovulate. If you think back to the Balanced Plate we've been talking about throughout this book, we need to make sure we're eating enough protein, fats, fibre and greens. If the thought of eating any of those foods fills you with fear, I strongly suggest you work with a nutritionist or nutritional therapist who has specific qualifications in eating disorders and disordered eating recovery.

If your period is missing or your menstrual cycles are irregular, there is hope. Whether you have PCOS or HA, it is possible to get your period back and have regular, stress-free menstrual cycles. As with other menstrual and reproductive health issues, it's essential that you take your recovery and treatment day by day, with a lot of patience and forgiveness for yourself.

CHAPTER 11
Thinking Beyond Your Period

Think about what you thought about your period when you started reading this book. Has anything changed? Hopefully, you've begun to see your period as part of a bigger picture: the four phases of your menstrual cycle, including ovulation. I've found that taking a more holistic view of my menstrual cycle has helped me to understand and anticipate the hormonal, physical, emotional and mental changes that take place during each phase.

It can take a while to be able to connect these changes with where you are in your menstrual cycle, but you'll get there. Try not to get frustrated if things aren't clicking right away.

If you're ever stuck, refer back to the chapter covering the phase you're currently in for a refresher, or check the tables on the next few pages for a quick summary.

The Four Phases of the Menstrual Cycle

Cycle Phase	Keywords	Biological	Physical	Hormonal	Mental and Social Effects
Menstrual Phase / Inner Winter	Surrender, rest, reflect	Your period begins and can last between 3–7 days	You may have less energy, you may experience light cramping, with mostly bright red blood throughout, your immune system may be slightly suppressed	Oestrogen and progesterone are at their lowest points, oestrogen starts to rise again around day 3 or 4, along with neurotransmitters like serotonin and dopamine	You may be less social, but more resilient, using this time to turn inward and evaluate different areas in your life, both big and small
Follicular Phase / Inner Spring	Play, energize, begin	The endometrium, or the lining of the uterus continues to grow and thicken	Your energy starts to increase, your skin may be clearer, and your hair thicker. Your libido begins to increase. Your cervical fluid gradually begins to thicken as a result of rising oestrogen.	FSH, oestrogen and testosterone continue to rise, with LH releasing in increasing pulse frequencies as you move closer to ovulation. Key brain neurotransmitters like serotonin, dopamine, acetylcholine and noradrenaline rise alongside oestrogen, contributing to increased confidence	You may start to feel more confident and social, open to newness and taking more risks in all areas of your life, with better communication skills

Ovulatory Phase / Inner Summer	Celebrate, dare, connect	The mature egg, or ovum, is released from one of your ovaries	Your energy is at its peak. You may experience *mittelschmerz*, or ovulation pain when the egg is released from the ovary. Your immune system is at its peak. Your cervical fluid changes, appearing like egg whites, and BBT rises just after ovulation to 36.4–37°C (97.5–98.6°F)	LH peaks and triggers ovulation. The corpus luteum releases progesterone and a second, smaller amount of oestrogen	You may feel at the peak of your powers, with strong communication and negotiation skills. Progesterone tamps down the wilder energy of the follicular phase to a calmer, more centred feeling
Luteal Phase / Inner Autumn	Slow down, organize, breathe	The endometrium continues to thicken. If the mature egg that was released during ovulation hasn't been fertilized, it starts to degrade and be absorbed into the endometrium, along with the corpus albicans	Your energy starts to gradually decline and you may notice changes in the appearance of your skin and breasts. Your BBT returns to pre-ovulatory levels	Oestrogen and progesterone gradually decline, returning to menstrual phase levels, along with neurotransmitters like serotonin, dopamine and acetylcholine	In the early luteal phase, you still feel the calming effects of progesterone. In the late luteal phase, declining hormones and neurotransmitters can increase self-doubt or self-criticism. You may have a greater need to organize, nest or get through your to-do list, powered by "get sh*t done" energy. Emotional resilience can decrease

What You Can Try During Each Phase

Cycle Phase	Nutrients and Food	Exercise / Movement	Lifestyle
Menstrual Phase / Inner Winter	**Iron:** grass-fed beef, lamb, dark poultry meat, chickpeas/ garbanzo beans, lentils, quinoa **Vitamin C:** citrus, kiwi, berries, broccoli, peppers **Copper:** organic beef liver, oysters, potatoes, mushrooms, dark / bittersweet chocolate **Magnesium:** Dark leafy greens, nuts, seeds **Zinc:** organic red meat, pumpkin, sunflower and sesame seeds, egg yolks, ginger, and organic dairy **Vitamin A:** beef liver, carrots, pumpkin, sweet potato, spinach, cod liver oil, spring/collard greens, kale **Vitamin B12:** organic red meat, dairy, eggs **Omega-3:** oily fish (SMASHHT), algae **Vitamin K:** natto (fermented soybeans), chard, organic beef or chicken liver, spring/collard greens, spinach, kale, broccoli	Slow flow yoga, restorative yoga, yin yoga, gentle swimming, walking	• Go a bit slower, if you can • Go to bed a bit earlier, take a longer bath and go into full self-care mode • Give yourself more time to get where you need to go and to get things done • Give yourself space to ponder something that's been on your mind • Use the box breathing exercise in Chapter 4 to help manage any pain or anxiety you might experience
Follicular Phase / Inner Spring	**Antioxidants:** citrus, almonds, leafy greens, brightly coloured fruits and vegetables **Selenium:** Brazil nuts, shellfish, pork **Zinc:** oysters, mussels, clams, pumpkin seeds **Choline:** eggs, free-range, organic meat and green vegetables such as broccoli and cauliflower **Fibre:** leafy greens, crucifers, nuts and seeds, fruit and vegetables with the peel on, carrots, sweet potato, quinoa, brown rice, brown pasta, brown bread **Phytoestrogens:** flax, miso, fermented tofu, natto, tempeh,	HIIT with a strength element Strong yoga, such as *ashtanga* or *vinyasa* flow, resistance training, Pilates	• Harness your energy so that you are using the energy of this phase wisely. Resist the urge to go all out • Try something new! • Schedule a big talk or presentation in this phase • Use the golden thread breathing exercise (page 133) to help harness energy • Find a focus for the increased sexual

Ovulatory Phase / Inner Summer	**Vitamin E:** sunflower seeds, almonds, avocados, kiwi, hazelnuts, spinach, chard **Vitamin B6:** wild salmon, chicken, sweet potato, avocados, banana, jackfruit **Vitamin D:** wild salmon, mushrooms, mackerel, canned salmon, milk, eggs **Probiotic food and drink:** kimchi, sauerkraut, pickled vegetables, fermented soy such as tofu, miso and tempeh, full-fat Greek or plain yogurt, kefir, kombucha	Anything that helps you take advantage of the ovulatory peak of energy Endurance exercise such as long runs, cycles or swims	• Continue to harness your energy so that you are using the energy of this phase wisely – try not to overschedule yourself! • Be social and connect with others • Pitch for new business, schedule your performance review or have a conversation with your mentor • Use the progressive muscle scan to help reduce cortisol levels and manage stress
Luteal Phase / Inner Autumn	**Increased protein and healthy fats** **Tryptophan:** poultry, red meat, pork, salmon, beans, pumpkin seeds, oats, eggs **Calcium:** sardines, salmon, full-fat yogurt, whole milk, cheese, tahini, spinach, black-eyed beans / peas, almonds **Potassium:** potatoes, apricots, prunes / dried plums, banana, artichokes, oranges, sunflower seeds, eggs **Iodine:** seaweed, cod, potatoes (especially the ones from Jersey!), prawns / shrimp, whole milk, eggs, tuna, strawberries	Listen to your body and do what feels right to you that day. Don't force it! Endurance exercise such as long runs, cycles or swims in the early luteal phase when progesterone is still high	• Slow down as you get further into the luteal phase • Harness the "get sh*t done" energy, but don't feel like you have to do everything! • Notice your mood and allow yourself to notice if any mood changes are the result of external events or if they're the result of hormonal changes

Tracking Your Menstrual Cycle

If you're not sure where to start, try tracking your menstrual cycle. This is a fantastic way to understand how everything I covered in this book applies to you and your body. This also helps you spot patterns and trends during successive menstrual cycles. You might notice that you get certain cravings on the day before your period, or you have a burst of creativity a few days before you ovulate. Menstrual cycle tracking also helps identify symptoms, when they happen, how often and their levels of severity. You'll then be able to put this all together and take it with you for appointments with your doctor or other healthcare professionals. You'll want to take at least three cycles' worth of information and data. I hope you'll find it empowering to be able to speak fluently about your health and what you're experiencing. I'll talk more about preparing for appointments with healthcare professionals later in this chapter.

If you have very irregular periods, PCOS, hypothalamic amenorrhea or are going through perimenopause or menopause, you may want to explore lunar cycle tracking, which uses the phases of the moon as a way of tracking your energy and mood. For more on this, I recommend the book *Luna: Harness the Power of the Moon to Live Your Best Life* (2020) by Tamara Driessen.

Where do you start with menstrual cycle tracking?

Day 1 of your period is the first day of your menstrual cycle, so that's a great place to start. Otherwise, you can start today by noticing how you feel and thinking about where in your cycle you might be.

You can track as much or as little as you want: just the start and end dates of your period and when you ovulate to all the details of your period, moods, pain, cravings, energy, cervical fluid, etc. – or somewhere in between. You can use the table on page 292 as a starting point, or you can use a journal, an Excel spreadsheet, the Notes app on your phone or an app such as Moody Month and Flo. If you have an Apple watch, you can even track your cycle using that! We have so many options now and it's been wonderful to watch how technology in the femtech space has evolved over the past ten years. When working with clients, I recommend they try a few techniques and keep the one that feels right for them. Some of them only had the headspace to track the date their period started and ended and when they ovulated, while other clients were much more involved, finding apps that allowed them to track and record all the detail they wanted to cover.

We've talked about how the length of our menstrual cycle can vary by a few days each month and how if you experience this, it is completely normal. Ovulation is the same. If you use a period tracking app, do not rely on the app to tell you when you're ovulating, especially if you're trying to conceive. A study of over 600,000 women found that ovulation did not typically occur on day 14 and cycle length differences were found to be predominantly caused by differences in follicular phase length.[1]

There are a number of factors, which we talked about in Chapter 6, that can affect ovulation. You might get less sleep or be more stressed one menstrual cycle. You might get sick and travel across time zones. These can all affect when you ovulate in the next one to two menstrual cycles. I encourage you, instead of relying on your cycle tracking app, to rely on the signs your body gives you to indicate you're ovulating: the changes in cervical fluid, libido, cervical position and basal body temperature.

After a while, you may find that you don't need to rely on your app or tracking system as much. That was my experience. When I was trying to get to the bottom of the period pain I was experiencing, I was diligent about noting my symptoms, their severity and when they took place, along with detailing everything else that was happening during my menstrual cycle. After a while, as the pain lessened, I found that I was more in tune with my body and I could tell what cycle phase I was in and how to adjust my work, social life, exercise and meals accordingly. Nowadays, I note when my period starts and ends, how I feel, when I ovulate and that's it.

Track as much as you want. This shouldn't feel overwhelming – if it does, that's a sign to pull back and just note the basics of your period and menstrual cycle.

Cycle Day	Period (Y / N)	Flow (Light / Medium / Heavy)	Menstrual Blood Colour	Temperature	Mood	Pain (Y / N describe and rate)
1						
2						
3						
4						
5						
6						
7						
8						
9						
10						
11						
12						
13						
14						
15						
16						
17						
18						
19						
20						
21						
22						
23						
24						
25						
26						
27						
28						
29						
30						
31						
32						
33						
34						
35						

Cravings	Energy (1–10)	Sleep	Cervical Fluid (Y / N, colour and thickness)	Any Other Symptoms?

Advocating for Yourself When Speaking with Medical Professionals

Going to the doctor's office can be an intimidating experience. You're thrust into a world with unfamiliar language and jargon, a time limit and a not-always-friendly face with whom you need to share intimate, personal information. Far too often, you might find yourself leaving the doctor's office feeling unheard and unclear about what you should do next.

I strongly encourage you to prepare for every appointment with your doctor and other healthcare professionals so that you can get the best possible outcome. I understand that this does put the onus on you, but when you only have ten minutes and can only focus on one issue, wouldn't you want to make the most of that time?

1. Ahead of the appointment, focus on the most important health issue and write down your related symptoms, when they happen, the levels of pain and quality of it, if any, and any other relevant information. Write down your questions and the outcome you would like. Would you like a referral or a specific test or investigation? Make you sure you note that down in your pre-appointment prep.
2. Know all your key information: menstrual cycle length and variations, length of your period, what ovulation and menstruation feel like for you.
3. Write everything down during the appointment so you can refer to it later, including the answers to your questions, referrals, treatments and investigations. You can also ask if you can record the discussion on your phone or tablet.
4. Don't be afraid to ask questions or get clarification on any medical jargon that's been used. This will help you leave your appointment with a full understanding of everything that's been said and the next steps.

5. Make sure everything has been noted in your NHS health records, including any refusals for tests, investigations and medication. This creates a paper trail that you can refer back to, especially if you change surgeries. At your new practice, they will request a copy of your health records from your previous doctor. You can also access your patient records online, including all test results, by registering for this service at your surgery.
6. If all of this feels really intimidating and you don't feel as though you can advocate for yourself, bring along a trusted friend or family member who can.

How To Have a Better Period (and Menstrual Cycle!)

When it comes to our periods and menstrual cycles, we're not aiming for perfection. I would simply like them to have less of a negative impact on your day-to-day life. I would love for you to get to a place where you don't dread the arrival of your period, where it doesn't dominate your life. You may not be ready to celebrate it, and if you do, that's a wonderful place to get to. You may not be ready to be period positive, to use the words of the body positivity movement. Could you get to a place of neutrality about your period: observing it when it arrives, noting how you feel, how it affects you and the shifts across the menstrual cycle?

If you take anything from this book, I hope it's these ten points.

1. Track your menstrual cycle and symptoms, if any
2. Have a bowel movement at least once a day
3. Drink enough water so that your pee is very light yellow
4. Eat your greens (and the rest of the veggies!)
5. Eat enough fat, protein and fibre in each meal
6. Get at least seven hours of sleep each night
7. Take a deep breath – our breath is one of our superpowers!

8. Move your body and get sweaty at least four times a week
9. Have regular orgasms
10. Find your community and nurture the connections with people that make you feel heard and vice versa

Thank you for reading this book. I hope that the information I've shared helps you have a better period, understand your menstrual cycle and tune into your body. Come find me on Instagram on @eatlovemove, use the hashtag #youcanhaveabetterperiod and let me know how you're getting on! Remember: you *can* have a better period!

Resources

Menstrual Health

Books
Beyond the Pill: A 30-day Program to Balance Your Hormones, Reclaim Your Body and Reverse the Dangerous Side Effects of the Birth Control Pill by Dr Jolene Brighten

Fix Your Period: Six Weeks to Life Long Hormone Balance by Nicole Jardim

Hormone Intelligence: The Complete Guide to Calming Hormone Chaos and Restoring Your Body's Natural Blueprint for Wellbeing by Dr Aviva Romm

Hormone Repair Manual: Every Woman's Guide to Healthy Hormones After 40 by Dr Lara Briden

How the Pill Changes Everything: Your Brain on Birth Control by Dr Sarah E. Hill

In the FLO: A 28-day Plan Working with Your Monthly Cycle to Do More and Stress Less by Alisa Vitti

Pain and Prejudice: A Call to Arms for Women and Their Bodies by Gabrielle Jackson

Period Power: Harness Your Hormones and Get Your Cycle Working for You by Maisie Hill

Period Repair Manual: Natural Treatment for Better Hormones and Better Periods by Dr Lara Briden

Taking Charge of Your Fertility: The Definitive Guide to Natural Birth Control, Pregnancy Achievement and Reproductive Health by Toni Weschler

The Balance Plan: Six Steps to Optimise Your Hormonal Health by Angelique Panagos

The Fifth Vital Sign: Master Your Cycles and Optimise Your Fertility by Lisa Hendrickson-Jack

The Hormone Cure: Reclaim Balance, Sleep and Sex Drive; Lose Weight; Feel Focused, Vital, and Energized Naturally with the Gottfried Protocol by Dr Sara Gottfried

Wild Power: Discover The Magic of Your Menstrual Cycle and Awaken the Feminine Path to Power by Alexandra Pope and Sjanie Hugo Wurlitzer

Womancode: Perfect Your Cycle, Amplify Your Fertility, Supercharge Your Sex Drive and Become a Power Source by Alisa Vitti

Websites
Dr Jolene Brighten: drbrighten.com
Dr Sara Gottfried: saragottfriedmd.com
Dr Aviva Romm: avivaromm.com
Lara Briden: larabriden.com
Nicole Jardim: nicolejardim.com

Podcasts
Period Story
Natural MD Radio
Fertility Friday
Period Party

Endometriosis

Books
Know Your Endo by Jessica Murnane
Outsmart Endometriosis by Dr Jessica Drummond
The Doctor Will See You Now by Dr Tamer Seckin

Websites
Endometriosis UK: www.endometriosis-uk.org
Endometriosis.net
Endo Black: endoblack.org

Know Your Endo: knowyourendo.com
QENDO: qendo.org.au

Adenomyosis

Books
Adenomyosis: A Significantly Neglected and Misunderstood Uterine Disorder by Maria Yeager

Fibroids

Books
Five Pounds of Fibroids: A Memoir by Rose Marie Johnson
Healing Fibroids: A Doctor's Natural Cure by Allan Warshowsky and Elena Ourmano
Uterine Fibroids: A Complete Guide by Elizabeth A. Stewart, MD

Websites
Fibroid Foundation: fibroidshealth.org

PMDD

Books
PMDD – A Guide to Coping With Pre-Menstrual Dysphoric Disorder by James E. Huston, MD and Lani C. Fujitsobo, PhD

Websites
International Association for Premenstrual Disorders: iapmd.org
Vicious Cycle PMDD: viciouscyclepmdd.com

PCOS

Books
8 Steps to Reverse Your PCOS by Dr Fiona McCulloch
Healing PCOS by Amy Medling
Natural Solutions to PCOS by Marilyn Glenville PhD

Websites
Verity: verity-pcos.org.uk
PCOS Awareness Association: pcosaa.org
Cysters: cysters.org

Hypothalamic Amenorrhea (HA)
No Period. Now What? A Guide to Regaining Your Cycles and Improving Your Fertility by Dr Nicola J. Rinaldi

Websites
BEAT: beateatingdisorders.org.uk
ANAD: anad.org

Other Resources

Stress
A Manual for Being Human by Dr Sophie Mort

Fatphobia
Fearing the Black Body: The Racial Origins of Fat Phobia by Sabrina Strings

Habits
Atomic Habits by James Clear
The Power of Habit: Why We Do What We Do and How to Change by Charles Duhigg
Tiny Habits by B.J. Fogg

Mindful Drinking
Drink: The Intimate Relationship Between Women and Alcohol by Ann Dowsett Johnson
Drink: The New Science of Alcohol and Health by Professor David Nutt
Love Yourself Sober: A Self-Care Guide to Alcohol Living for Busy Mothers by Kate Baily and Mandy Manners
Mindful Drinking: How Cutting Down Can Change Your Life by Rosamund Dean

Desire
Come as You Are: The Surprising New Science That Will Transform Your Sex Life by Dr Emily Nagoski

CBD
The CBD Bible by Dr Dani Gordon

The Moon
Luna: Harness the Power of the Moon to Live Your Best Life by Tamara Driessen

Hormone-friendly Swaps

Make-up, skincare and haircare
contentbeautywellbeing.com, naturisimo.com and theafrohairandskincarecompany.co.uk are fantastic websites with a wide variety of natural and organic beauty and haircare products.

Soap
Faith in Nature, Jason, Dr Bronner

Toothpaste
Jason, Dr Bronner, Georganics, Kingfisher, Kurin, RiseWell, Organic People

Deodorant
Wild, The Natural Deodorant Co., Native Unearthed

Menstrual products
unfabled.co is a great one-stop shop for menstrual products

Period underwear
Flux, Wuka, Modibodi, M&S, Knix, Hey Girls, Thinx

Menstrual cups
TOTM, Lunette, Saalt, &SISTERS, Mooncup, OrganicCup, Athena, Hey Girls, Diva Cup

Reusable and disposable pads
Natracare, Bloom and Nora, Wear 'Em Out, &SISTERS, Flo, Organyc, Yoni, Hey Girls, Honour Your Flow, The Eco Woman, Grace & Green

Tampons
Daye, TOTM, &SISTERS, Freda, Dame, Yoni, Hey Girls

Cleaning and laundry products
Ecover, Attitude, Ecozone, Spruce, Dr Bronner, Clara

Acknowledgements

I'm so grateful to everyone that has supported me on my writing journey. It's been a long-time dream to write this book and get more information out there about how to have a better period and menstrual cycle. I'm so thrilled my words are in your hands!

To the whole Watkins team who helped bring this book to life – I'm so thankful for your support. Anya – thank you for believing in me when I didn't believe in myself, for chasing me when I was procrastinating and helping to shape my words. Fiona, Brittany and Meredith – thank you for taking this book over the finishing line with tough but necessary editing. Your supports means a lot. Laura, Isabelle, Lauren and Rachel – thank you for your megaphone and letting people know about this book. Sneha – thank you for the beautiful illustrations. Glen – you took my ideas and designed a brilliant cover. Steve and Uzma – thank you for translating my notes into a fantastic-looking book, both inside and out.

To my agent, Laura McNeill. You took a chance on me, you fought my corner and your notes made this book infinitely better. I appreciate you. To Megan and the rest of the Gleam team, thank you.

To all my clients – thank you for trusting me to help you improve your menstrual and hormone health.

To my podcast guests – thank you for your openness and trusting me with your stories. By sharing your experiences, you've helped to begin to break menstrual health taboos.

To my friends and family – sorry for disappearing while I was in my writing cave. Your support and nudges to keep going when I was frustrated and procrastinating helped to push me over the finish line.

And most of all, to M & J. I love you both so much.

About the Author

Le'Nise Brothers is the author of *You Can Have a Better Period*.

Le'Nise is a registered nutritionist, specializing in women's health, hormones and the menstrual cycle. She is a member of the British Association of Nutritional Therapists (BANT) and the Complementary and Natural Health Council (CNHC). She is also a yoga teacher and host of the Period Story podcast.

Le'Nise studied at the College of Naturopathic Medicine and is the founder of the nutrition and wellbeing practice Eat Love Move.

She is a passionate and knowledgeable public speaker who believes our menstrual cycle is one of our superpowers and that we all deserve better menstrual health. Her work is influenced by her own experience and those of the many women she's helped to improve their menstrual and hormone health through her private practice, group programmes, talks and workshops.

Le'Nise is originally from Canada and now lives in London, England with her husband and son.

Ways to connect with Le'Nise:
Website: www.eatlovemove.com
[Instagram] @eatlovemove
[Facebook] @eatlovemovenutrition
Podcast: Period Story

Notes

Introduction
1 NHS, "Period Pain", 2019. nhs.uk/conditions/period-pain/

Chapter 1
1 instagram.com/p/CNiJGT8nYI3/
2 Caplan, P., "The Strange Case of Dr. Jekyll and Ms. Hyde: How PMS became a cultural phenomenon and a psychiatric disorder", *Annual Review of Sex Research*, 2002; 13(1), p.276
3 Wenger, B., "Mikveh", *The Shalvi / Hyman Encyclopedia of Jewish Women*, 2019. jwa.org/encyclopedia/article/mikveh/
4 Singh, N.-G.K., *The Feminine Principle in the Sikh Vision of the Transcendent*, Cambridge University Press, 2008, p.4
5 Adhikari, R., "Bringing an end to deadly 'menstrual huts' is proving difficult in Nepal", *BMJ*, 2012; 368(8234). bmj.com/content/368/bmj.m536
6 Amatya, P., Ghimire, S., Callahan, K.E., Baral, B.K. and Poudel, K.C., "Practice and lived experience of menstrual exiles (Chhaupadi) among adolescent girls in far-western Nepal", *PLOS One*, 2018; 13(12), p.e0208260
7 Adhikari, R., "Destroy 'period huts' or forget state support: Nepal moves to end practice", *Guardian*, 14 January 2019. theguardian.com/global-development/2019/jan/14/destroy-period-huts-or-forget-state-support-nepal-moves-to-end-practice-chhaupadi
8 Mukherjee, A., Lama, M., Khakurel, U., Jha, A.N., Ajose, F., Acharya, S., Tymes-Wilbekin, K., Sommer, M., Jolly, P.E., Lhaki, P. and Shrestha, S., "Perception and practices of menstruation restrictions among urban adolescent girls and women in Nepal: A cross-sectional survey", *Reproductive Health*, 2020; 17(1), p.2
9 Hennegan, J., Shannon, A.K., Rubli, J., Schwab, K.J. and Melendez-Torres, G.J., "Women's and girls' experiences of menstruation in low- and middle-income countries: A systematic review and qualitative metasynthesis", *PLOS Medicine*, 2019; 16(5). ncbi.nlm.nih.gov/pmc/articles/PMC6521998/
10 Genesis 3:16, *Bible Gateway*, n.d., biblegateway.com/verse/en/Genesis%203:16]

11 Pliny the Elder, "Facts connected to the menstrual discharge", *The Natural History, Book XXVII: Remedies Derived from Living Creatures*. perseus.tufts.edu/hopper/text?doc=Perseus%3Atext%3A1999.02.0137%3Abook%3D28%3Achapter%3D23

12 Markstrom, C.A., *Empowerment of North American Indian Girls: Ritual Expressions at Puberty*, University of Nebraska Press, 2010, pp.192–193

13 Upadhyay, P., पीरियड्स: दक्षिण भारत मे शर्म नही जश्न है पहला पीरियड, *Firstpost Hindi*, 2018. hindi.firstpost.com/special/periods-are-not-shame-but-festival-in-south-india-first-period-ritu-kala-samskara-or-half-saree-festival-is-well-known-pad-man-akshay-kumar-and-radhika-apte-87227.html

Chapter 2

1 American College of Obstetricians and Gynecologists, "Menstruation in girls and adolescents: Using the menstrual cycle as a vital sign", *Obstet Gynecol*, 2015; 651. acog.org/clinical/clinical-guidance/committee-opinion/articles/2015/12/menstruation-in-girls-and-adolescents-using-the-menstrual-cycle-as-a-vital-sign

Chapter 3

1 Strings, S., *Fearing The Black Body: The Racial Origins of Fat Phobia*, New York University Press, 2019, pp.187 –200

2 Ibid.

3 World Health Organization, "Body mass index – BMI", euro.who.int/en/health-topics/disease-prevention/nutrition/a-healthy-lifestyle/body-mass-index-bmi

4 Dusenbery, M., *Doing Harm: The Truth About How Bad Medicine And Lazy Science Leave Women Dismissed, Misdiagnosed, And Sick*, Harper One, 2019, pp.137–171

5 Crawford, R., "Healthism and the medicalization of everyday life", *International Journal of Health Services*, 1980; 10(3), pp.365–388

6 Akinrodoye, M.A. and Lui, F., "Neuroanatomy, somatic nervous system", *PubMed, StatPearls Publishing*, 2020. ncbi.nlm.nih.gov/books/NBK556027/

7 Volpi, E., Nazemi, R. and Fujita, S., "Muscle tissue changes with aging", *Current Opinion in Clinical Nutrition and Metabolic Care*, 2004; 7(4), pp.405–10. ncbi.nlm.nih.gov/pmc/articles/PMC2804956/

8 Jenkins, T., Nguyen, J., Polglaze, K. and Bertrand, P., "Influence of tryptophan and serotonin on mood and cognition with a possible role of the gut-brain axis", *Nutrients*, 2016; 8(1), p.56. ncbi.nlm.nih.gov/pmc/articles/PMC4728667/

9 Fernstrom, J.D. and Fernstrom, M.H., "Tyrosine, phenylalanine, and catecholamine synthesis and function in the brain", *Journal of Nutrition*, 2007; 137(6), pp.1539S–1547S

10 Rousset, B., Dupuy, C., Miot, F. and Dumont, J., "Chapter 2: Thyroid hormone synthesis and secretion", in Feingold, K.R. et al (eds), *Endotext, MDText.com,* 2015. ncbi.nlm.nih.gov/books/NBK285550/

11 Gorczyca, A.M., Sjaarda, L.A., Mitchell, E.M., Perkins, N.J., Schliep, K.C., Wactawski-Wende, J. and Mumford, S.L., "Changes in macronutrient, micronutrient, and food group intakes throughout the menstrual cycle in healthy, premenopausal women", *European Journal of Nutrition,* 2015; 55(3), pp.1181–1188

12 Maljaars, J., Romeyn, E.A., Haddeman, E., Peters, H.P. and Masclee, A.A., "Effect of fat saturation on satiety, hormone release, and food intake", *American Journal of Clinical Nutrition,* 2009; 89(4), pp.1019–1024. academic.oup.com/ajcn/article/89/4/1019/4596700

13 Holst, J.P., Soldin, O.P., Guo, T. and Soldin, S.J., "Steroid hormones: Relevance and measurement in the clinical laboratory", *Clinics in Laboratory Medicine,* 2004; 24(1), pp.105–118. ncbi.nlm.nih.gov/pmc/articles/PMC3636985/

14 Hu, J., Zhang, Z., Shen, W.-J. and Azhar, S., "Cellular cholesterol delivery, intracellular processing and utilization for biosynthesis of steroid hormones", *Nutrition & Metabolism,* 2010; 7(1), p.47

15 De Souza, R.J., Mente, A., Maroleanu, A., Cozma, A.I., Ha, V., Kishibe, T., Uleryk, E., Budylowski, P., Schünemann, H., Beyene, J. and Anand, S.S., "Intake of saturated and trans unsaturated fatty acids and risk of all cause mortality, cardiovascular disease, and type 2 diabetes: Systematic review and meta-analysis of observational studies", *BMJ,* 2015; 351, p.h3978. bmj.com/content/351/bmj.h3978

16 Draper, C.F., Duisters, K., Weger, B., Chakrabarti, A., Harms, A.C., Brennan, L., Hankemeier, T., Goulet, L., Konz, T., Martin, F.P., Moco, S. and van der Greef, J., "Menstrual cycle rhythmicity: Metabolic patterns in healthy women", *Scientific Reports,* 2018; 8. ncbi.nlm.nih.gov/pmc/articles/PMC6167362/

17 Hodges, R.E. and Minich, D.M., "Modulation of metabolic detoxification pathways using foods and food-derived components: A scientific review with clinical application", *Journal of Nutrition and Metabolism,* 2015 (760689), pp.1–23. ncbi.nlm.nih.gov/pmc/articles/PMC4488002/

18 Higdon, J., Delage, B., Williams, D. and Dashwood, R., "Cruciferous vegetables and human cancer risk: Epidemiologic evidence and mechanistic basis", *Pharmacological Research,* 2007; 55(3), pp.224–236

19 McRae, M.P., "Dietary fiber intake and type 2 diabetes mellitus: An umbrella review of meta-analyses", *Journal of Chiropractic Medicine,* 2018; 17(1), pp.44–53

20 Silva, Y.P., Bernardi, A. and Frozza, R.L., "The role of short-chain fatty acids from gut microbiota in gut-brain communication", *Frontiers in Endocrinology,* 2020; 11(25), pp.2–5

21 NHS Choices, "How to get more fibre into your diet", 2018. nhs.uk/live-well/eat-well/how-to-get-more-fibre-into-your-diet/

22 Pavan, R., Jain, S., Shraddha and Kumar, A., "Properties and therapeutic application of bromelain: A review", *Biotechnology Research International*, 2012, pp.1–6

23 Maskarinec, G., Beckford, F., Morimoto, Y., Franke, A.A. and Stanczyk, F.Z., "Association of estrogen measurements in serum and urine of premenopausal women", *Biomarkers in Medicine*, 2015; 9(5), pp.417–424

24 Silva, J.F., Ocarino, N.M. and Serakides, R., "Thyroid hormones and female reproduction", *Biology of Reproduction*, 2018; 99(5), p.907

25 Santin, A.P. and Furlanetto, T.W., "Role of estrogen in thyroid function and growth regulation", *Journal of Thyroid Research*, 2011, pp.1–7

26 Vigil, P., Lyon, C., Flores, B., Rioseco, H. and Serrano, F., "Ovulation, a sign of health", *Linacre Quarterly*, 2017; 84(4), pp.343–355. ncbi.nlm.nih.gov/pmc/articles/PMC5730019/

27 Chiovato, L., Magri, F. and Carlé, A., "Hypothyroidism in context: Where we've been and where we're going", *Advances in Therapy*, 2019; 36(Suppl 2), pp.47–58. ncbi.nlm.nih.gov/pmc/articles/PMC6822815/

28 Gurgul, E. and Sowiński, J., "Primary hyperthyroidism — diagnosis and treatment: Indications and contraindications for radioiodine therapy", *Nuclear Medicine Review*, 2011; 14(1), pp.29–32

29 Philippe, J. and Dibner, C., "Thyroid circadian timing", *Journal of Biological Rhythms*, 2014; 30(2), pp.76–83

Chapter 4

1   Ofojekwu, M.-J.N., Nnanna, O.U., Okolie, C.E., Odewumi, L.A., Isiguzoro, I.O.U. and Lugos, M.D., "Hemoglobin and serum iron concentrations in menstruating nulliparous women in Jos, Nigeria", *Laboratory Medicine*, 2013; 44(2), pp.121–124. academic.oup.com/labmed/article/44/2/121/2657721

2   Pahwa, R., Goyal, A., Bansal, P. and Jialal, I., "Chronic Inflammation", *Statpearls*, 2019, ncbi.nlm.nih.gov/books/NBK493173/

3   Cederbaum, A.I., "Alcohol metabolism", *Clinics in Liver Disease*, 2012; 16(4), pp.667–685. ncbi.nlm.nih.gov/pmc/articles/PMC3484320/

4   Herman-Giddens, M.E., "The decline in the age of menarche in the United States: Should we be concerned?", *Journal of Adolescent Health*, 2007; 40(3), pp. 201–203, 10.1016/j.jadohealth.2006.12.019

5   NHS, "Early or Delayed Puberty", 3 Oct. 2018. nhs.uk/conditions/early-or-delayed-puberty/

6   Committee on Adolescent Health Care, "Menstruation in girls and adolescents: Using the menstrual cycle as a vital sign", *Acog.org*, 2015, acog.org/clinical/clinical-guidance/committee-opinion/articles/2015/12/menstruation-in-girls-and-adolescents-using-the-menstrual-cycle-as-a-vital-sign

7 Malgorzata, D., Malgorzata, G. and Tabarowski, K.-S.M. and Z., "The primordial to primary follicle transition: A reliable marker of ovarian function", *Insights from Animal Reproduction*, 2016. intechopen.com/books/insights-from-animal-reproduction/the-primordial-to-primary-follicle-transition-a-reliable-marker-of-ovarian-function

8 Hannon, P.R. and Curry, T.E., "Folliculogenesis", *Encyclopedia of Reproduction*, Elsevier, 2018, pp. 72–79

9 Ibid.

10 Pahwa, R., Goyal, A., Bansal, P. and Jialal, I., "Chronic Inflammation", *Statpearls*, 2019, ncbi.nlm.nih.gov/books/NBK493173/

11 Thiyagarajan, D.K. et al, "Physiology, menstrual cycle", *StatPearls*, 2021. ncbi.nlm.nih.gov/books/NBK500020/#article-24987.s4

12 Hill, S.E., *How the Pill Changes Everything: Your Brain on Birth Control*, Orion Spring, 2019

13 Miro, F. and Aspinall, L.J., "The onset of the initial rise in follicle-stimulating hormone during the human menstrual cycle", *Human Reproduction*, 2005; 20(1), pp.96–100. 10.1093/humrep/deh551

14 Reed, B.G., and Carr, B.R., "The normal menstrual cycle and the control of ovulation", *MDText.com, Inc.*, 5 August 2018. ncbi.nlm.nih.gov/books/NBK279054/

15 Ibid.

16 Delgado, B.J. and Lopez-Ojeda, W., "Estrogen", *StatPearls*, 3 October 2019. ncbi.nlm.nih.gov/books/NBK538260/

17 Rybaczyk, L.A. et al, "An overlooked connection: Serotonergic mediation of estrogen-related physiology and pathology", *BMC Women's Health*, 2005; 5(1). ncbi.nlm.nih.gov/pmc/articles/PMC1327664/

18 Ibid.

19 Bethea, C.L. et al, "Steroid regulation of tryptophan hydroxylase protein in the dorsal raphe of macaques", *Biological Psychiatry*, 2000; 47(6), pp.562–576. 10.1016/s0006-3223(99)00156-0

20 Hernández-Hernández, O.T. et al, "Role of estradiol in the expression of genes involved in serotonin neurotransmission: Implications for female depression", *Current Neuropharmacology*, 2019; 17(5), pp.459–471. 10.2174/1570159x16666180628165107

21 Pope, A. and Wurlitzer. S.H., *Wild Power: Discover the Magic of Your Menstrual Cycle and Awaken the Feminine Path to Power*, Hay House, 2017

22 Barth, C. et al, "Sex Hormones affect neurotransmitters and shape the adult female brain during hormonal transition periods", *Frontiers in Neuroscience*, 2015; 9(37). 10.3389/fnins.2015.00037

23 Maki, P.M. et al, "Implicit memory varies across the menstrual cycle: Estrogen effects in young women", *Neuropsychologia*, 2002; 40(5), pp.518–529. 10.1016/s0028-3932(01)00126-9

24 Hausmann, M. et al, "Sex hormones affect spatial abilities during the menstrual cycle", *Behavioral Neuroscience*, 2000; 114(6), pp.1245–1250. 10.1037/0735-7044.114.6.1245

25 Thiyagarajan, D.K. et al, "Physiology, menstrual cycle", *StatPearls*, 2021. ncbi.nlm.nih.gov/books/NBK500020/#article-24987.s4

26 Jain, V. and Wotring, V.E., "Medically induced amenorrhea in female astronauts", *npj Microgravity*, 2016; 2(1), p.1

27 Holohan, M., "Do you get your period in space? Why microgravity menstruation matters", *TODAY.com*, 2016. today.com/health/do-you-get-your-period-in-space-why-microgravity-menstruation-matters-t87711.

28 Gupte, A.A., Pownall, H.J. and Hamilton, D.J., "Estrogen: An emerging regulator of insulin action and mitochondrial function", *Journal of Diabetes Research*, 2015 (916585), pp.1–9

29 Yeung, E.H., Zhang, C., Mumford, S.L., Ye, A., Trevisan, M., Chen, L., Browne, R.W., Wactawski-Wende, J. and Schisterman, E.F., "Longitudinal study of insulin resistance and sex hormones over the menstrual cycle: The biocycle study", *Journal of Clinical Endocrinology & Metabolism*, 2010; 95(12), pp.5435–5442

30 Napolitano, M. et al, "Iron-dependent erythropoiesis in women with excessive menstrual blood losses and women with normal menses", *Annals of Hematology*, 2013; 93(4), pp.557–563. 10.1007/s00277-013-1901-3

31 nhs.uk/conditions/iron-deficiency-anaemia/

32 NHS Choices, "Iron – vitamins and minerals", 2019. nhs.uk/conditions/vitamins-and-minerals/iron/

33 Doguer, C. et al, "Intersection of iron and copper metabolism in the mammalian intestine and liver", *Comprehensive Physiology*, 2018; 8(4), pp.1433–1461. 10.1002/cphy.c170045

34 Micronutrient Information Center, "Copper", Linus Pauling Institute, Oregon State University, 2014. lpi.oregonstate.edu/mic/minerals/copper

35 Hurrell, R. and Egli, ., "Iron bioavailability and dietary reference values", *American Journal of Clinical Nutrition*, 2010; 91(5), pp.1461S–1467S. 10.3945/ajcn.2010.28674f

36 US Department of Agriculture, Agriculture Research Service, *FoodData Central*, 2019. fdc.nal.usda.gov/index.html.

37 Ibid.

38 Ibid.

39 Ibid.

40 Broadley, M.R. and White, P.J., "Eats roots and leaves: Can edible horticultural crops address dietary calcium, magnesium and potassium deficiencies?", *Proceedings of the Nutrition Society*, 2010; 69(4), pp.601–612. 10.1017/s0029665110001588

41 Office of Dietary Supplements, "Magnesium", *National Institutes of Health*, 2015. ods.od.nih.gov/factsheets/Magnesium-HealthProfessional/#h5

42 Rosanoff, A., Weaver, C.M. and Rude, R.K., "Suboptimal magnesium status in the United States: Are the health consequences underestimated?", *Nutrition Reviews*, 2012; 70(3), pp.153–164

43 US Department of Agriculture, Agriculture Research Service, *FoodData Central, 2019.* fdc.nal.usda.gov/index.html

44 Al-Mekhlafi, H.M., Al-Zabedi, E.M., Al-Maktari, M.T., Atroosh, W.M., Al-Delaimy, A.K., Moktar, N., Sallam, A.A., Abdullah, W.A., Jani, R. and Surin, J., "Effects of vitamin A supplementation on iron status indices and iron deficiency anaemia: A randomized controlled trial", *Nutrients*, 2013; 6(1), pp.190–206. ncbi.nlm.nih.gov/pmc/articles/PMC3916855/

45 Office of Dietary Supplements, "Vitamin A", *National Institutes of Health*, 2012. ods.od.nih.gov/factsheets/VitaminA-HealthProfessional

46 Bastos Maia, S., Rolland Souza, A., Costa Caminha, M., Lins da Silva, S., Callou Cruz, R., Carvalho dos Santos, C. and Batista Filho, M., "Vitamin A and pregnancy: A narrative review", *Nutrients*, 2019; 11(3), p.681

47 US Department of Agriculture, Agriculture Research Service, *FoodData Central*, 2019. fdc.nal.usda.gov/index.html.

48 Ibid

49 Micronutrient Information Center, "Vitamin B12", Linus Pauling Institute, Oregon State University, 22 April 2014, lpi.oregonstate.edu/mic/vitamins/vitamin-B12

50 US Department of Agriculture, Agriculture Research Service, *FoodData Central*, 2019. fdc.nal.usda.gov/index.html.

51 Rahbar, N., Asgharzadeh, N. and Ghorbani, R., "Effect of omega-3 fatty acids on intensity of primary dysmenorrhea", *International Journal of Gynecology & Obstetrics*, 2012; 117(1), pp.45–47

52 Zafari, M., Behmanesh, F. and Agha Mohammadi, A., "Comparison of the effect of fish oil and ibuprofen on treatment of severe pain in primary dysmenorrhea", *Caspian Journal of Internal Medicine*, 2011; 2(3), pp.279–282

53 Office of Dietary Supplements, "Omega-3 Fatty Acids", *National Institutes of Health*, 2017. ods.od.nih.gov/factsheets/Omega3FattyAcids-HealthProfessional/

54 US Department of Agriculture, Agriculture Research Service, *FoodData Central*, 2019. fdc.nal.usda.gov/index.html.

55 Johnson, L.E., "Vitamin K Deficiency", *MSD Manual Professional Edition*, 2020. msdmanuals.com/en-gb/professional/nutritional-disorders/vitamin-deficiency-dependency-and-toxicity/vitamin-k-deficiency

56 Micronutrient Information Center, "Vitamin K", Linus Pauling Institute, Oregon State University, 5 August 2019. lpi.oregonstate.edu/mic/vitamins/vitamin-K

57 US Department of Agriculture, Agriculture Research Service, *FoodData Central*, 2019. fdc.nal.usda.gov/index.html.

58 Bruinvels, G. et al, "The prevalence and impact of heavy menstrual bleeding (menorrhagia) in elite and non-elite athletes", *PLOS One*, 2016; 11(2), p.e0149881. ncbi.nlm.nih.gov/pmc/articles/PMC4763330/, 10.1371/journal.pone.0149881

59 Slauterbeck, J.R., Fuzie, S.F., Smith, M.P., Clark, R.J., Xu, K., Starch, D.W. and Hardy, D.M., "The menstrual cycle, sex hormones, and anterior cruciate ligament injury", *Journal of athletic training*, 2012; 37(3), pp.275–278. ncbi.nlm.nih.gov/pmc/articles/PMC164356/

Chapter 5

1 Fehring, R.J. et al, "Variability in the phases of the menstrual cycle", *Journal of Obstetric, Gynecologic & Neonatal Nursing*, 2006; 35(3), pp.376–384. 10.1111/j.1552-6909.2006.00051.x

2 Vigil, P., Lyon, C., Flores, B., Rioseco, H. and Serrano, F., "Ovulation: A sign of health", *Linacre Quarterly*, 2017; 84(4), pp.343–355. ncbi.nlm.nih.gov/pmc/articles/PMC5730019 /

3 The vaginal pH changes as we get closer to ovulation, becoming more alkaline and helping the vagina become more hospitable to sperm. It is usually acidic, with a low pH that protects the vagina. This is the reason dark or black underwear can look bleached or faded, a fact I only learned in the past year, having spent years thinking something was wrong with me. If you're in the same boat, this just means you have a healthy vagina!

4 Sakkas, D., Ramalingam, M., Garrido, N. and Barratt, C.L.R., "Sperm selection in natural conception: What can we learn from Mother Nature to improve assisted reproduction outcomes?", *Human Reproduction Update*, 2015; 21(6), pp.711–726. ncbi.nlm.nih.gov/pmc/articles/PMC4594619/

5 Su, H.-W., Yi, Y.-C., Wei, T.-Y., Chang, T.-C. and Cheng, C.-M., "Detection of ovulation: A review of currently available methods", *Bioengineering & Translational Medicine*, 2017; 2(3), pp.238–246

6 Herbison, A.E., "A simple model of estrous cycle negative and positive feedback regulation of GnRH secretion", *Frontiers in Neuroendocrinology*, 2012, 57, p.100837

7 Thompson, I.R. and Kaiser, U.B., "GnRH pulse frequency-dependent differential regulation of LH and FSH gene expression", *Molecular and Cellular Endocrinology*, 2014; 385(1–2), pp.28–35. ncbi.nlm.nih.gov/pmc/articles/PMC3947649 /

8 Orlowski, M. and Sarao, M.S., "Physiology, follicle stimulating hormone", *National Institutes of Health*, 2018. ncbi.nlm.nih.gov/books/NBK535442/

9 Reed, B.G., and Carr, B.R., "The normal menstrual cycle and the control of ovulation", *MDText.com, Inc.*, 5 August 2018. ncbi.nlm.nih.gov/books/NBK279054/

10 Raghunath, R.S., Venables, Z.C. and Millington, G.W.M., "The menstrual cycle and the skin", *Clinical and Experimental Dermatology*, 2015; 40(2), pp.111–115

11 Oertelt-Prigione, S., "Immunology and the menstrual cycle", *Autoimmunity reviews*, 2012; 11(6-7), pp.A486–92. ncbi.nlm.nih.gov/pubmed/22155200

12 Cappelletti, M. and Wallen, K., "Increasing women's sexual desire: The comparative effectiveness of estrogens and androgens", *Hormones and Behavior*, 2016; 78, pp.178–193. ncbi.nlm.nih.gov/pmc/articles/PMC4720522 /

13 Thiyagarajan, D.K. et al, "Physiology, menstrual cycle", *StatPearls*, 2021. ncbi.nlm.nih.gov/books/NBK500020/#article-24987.s4

14 Boudesseul, J. et al, "Do women expose themselves to more health-related risks in certain phases of the menstrual cycle? A meta-analytic review". *Neuroscience & Biobehavioral Reviews*, 2019; 107, pp.505–524. 10.1016/j.neubiorev.2019.08.016

15 Hidalgo-Lopez, E. and Pletzer, B., "Interactive effects of dopamine baseline levels and cycle phase on executive functions: The role of progesterone", *Frontiers in Neuroscience*, 2017, 11, p.2

16 Bauer, J.L., Kuhn, K., Al-Safi, Z., Harris, M.A., Eckel, R.H., Bradford, A.P., Robledo, C.Y., Malkhasyan, A., Gee, N. and Polotsky, A.J., "Omega-3 fatty acid supplementation significantly lowers FSH in young normal weight women", *Fertility and Sterility*, 2017; 108(3), pp.e257–e258

17 Qazi, I., Angel, C., Yang, H., Pan, B., Zoidis, E., Zeng, C.-J., Han, H. and Zhou, G.-B., "Selenium, selenoproteins, and female reproduction: A review", *Molecules*, 2018; 23(12), p.3053

18 Micronutrient Information Center, "Selenium", Linus Pauling Institute, Oregon State University, 2019. lpi.oregonstate.edu/mic/minerals/selenium

19 Pandey, K.B. and Rizvi, S.I., "Plant polyphenols as dietary antioxidants in human health and disease", *Oxidative Medicine and Cellular Longevity*, 2009; 2(5), pp.270–278. ncbi.nlm.nih.gov/pmc/articles/PMC2835915/

20 Bedwal, R.S. and Bahuguna, A., "Zinc, copper and selenium in reproduction", *Experientia*, 1994; 50(7), pp.626–640

21 Office of Dietary Supplements, "Zinc", *National Institutes of Health*, 2021, ods.od.nih.gov/factsheets/Zinc-HealthProfessional/#h5

22 US Department of Agriculture, Agriculture Research Service, *FoodData Central*, 2019. fdc.nal.usda.gov/index.html.

23 Schlemmer, U., Frølich, W., Prieto, R.M. and Grases, F., "Phytate in foods and significance for humans: Food sources, intake, processing, bioavailability, protective role and analysis", *Molecular Nutrition & Food Research*, 2009; 53(S2), pp.S330–S375

24 Korsmo, H.W., Jiang, X. and Caudill, M.A., "Choline: Exploring the growing science on its benefits for moms and babies", *Nutrients*, 2019; 11(8), p.1823. ncbi.nlm.nih.gov/pmc/articles/PMC6722688/

25 Micronutrient Information Center, "Choline", Linus Pauling Institute, Oregon State University, 2014. lpi.oregonstate.edu/mic/other-nutrients/choline

26 US Department of Agriculture, Agriculture Research Service, *FoodData Central*, 2019. fdc.nal.usda.gov/index.html.

27 Dikeman, C.L. and Fahey, G.C., "Viscosity as related to dietary fiber: A review", *Critical Reviews in Food Science and Nutrition*, 2006; 46(8), pp.649–663

28 Plottel, C.S. and Blaser, M.J., "Microbiome and malignancy", *Cell Host & Microbe*, 2011; 10(4), pp.324–335

29 Kwa, M., Plotell, C.S., Blaser, M.J. and Adams, S., "The Intestinal microbiome and estrogen receptor–positive female breast cancer", *Journal of the National Cancer Institute*, 2016; 108(8), p.3

30 Zhao, E. and Mu, Q., "Phytoestrogen biological actions on mammalian reproductive system and cancer growth", *Scientia Pharmaceutica*, 2011; 79(1), pp.1–20. ncbi.nlm.nih.gov/pmc/articles/PMC3097497/

31 Desmawati, D. and Sulastri, D., "A phytoestrogens and their health effect", *Open Access Macedonian Journal of Medical Sciences*, 2019; 7(3), pp.495–499

32 Mukherjee, R., Chakraborty, R. and Dutta, A., " Role of fermentation in improving nutritional quality of soybean meal: A review", *Asian-Australasian Journal of Animal Sciences*, 2016; 29(11), pp.1523–1529. ncbi.nlm.nih.gov/pmc/articles/PMC5088370/

Chapter 6

1 Black, L.E., Swan, P.D. and Alvar, B.A., "Effects of intensity and volume on insulin sensitivity during acute bouts of resistance training", *Journal of Strength and Conditioning Research*, 2010; 24(4), pp.1109–1116

2 Lambalk, C.B., Boomsma, D.I., de Boer, L., de Koning, C.H., Schoute, E., Popp-Snijders, C. and Schoemaker, J., "Increased levels and pulsatility of follicle-stimulating hormone in mothers of hereditary dizygotic twins", *Journal of Clinical Endocrinology & Metabolism*, 1998; 83(2), pp.481–486

3 Zinaman, M.J., "Using cervical mucus and other easily observed biomarkers to identify ovulation in prospective pregnancy trials", *Paediatric and Perinatal Epidemiology*, 2006; 20(s1), pp.26–29

4 Vigil, P., Lyon, C., Flores, B., Rioseco, H. and Serrano, F., "Ovulation: A sign of health", *Linacre Quarterly*, 2017; 84(4), pp.343–355. ncbi.nlm.nih.gov/pmc/articles/PMC5730019/

5   Weschler, T., *Taking charge of your fertility: The definitive guide to natural birth control, pregnancy achievement, and reproductive health; 20th Anniversary Edition,* William Morrow, 2015

6   Direito, A., Bailly, S., Mariani, A. and Ecochard, R., "Relationships between the luteinizing hormone surge and other characteristics of the menstrual cycle in normally ovulating women", *Fertility and Sterility,* 2013; 99(1), pp.279-285.e3

7   Prior, J., "Women's reproductive system as balanced estradiol and progesterone actions: A revolutionary, paradigm-shifting concept in women's health", *Drug Discovery Today: Disease Models,* 2020; 32(B), pp.31–40. sciencedirect.com/science/article/pii/S174067572030013X

8   Vigil, P., Lyon, C., Flores, B., Rioseco, H. and Serrano, F., "Ovulation: A sign of health", *Linacre Quarterly,* 2017; 84(4), pp.343–355. ncbi.nlm.nih.gov/pmc/articles/PMC5730019/

9   Mesen, T.B. and Young, S.L., "Progesterone and the luteal phase", *Obstetrics and Gynecology Clinics of North America,* 2015; 42(1), pp.135–151

10 Cable, J.K. and Grider, M.H., "Physiology, progesterone", *PubMed,* 2010. ncbi.nlm.nih.gov/books/NBK558960/

11 Taraborrelli, S., "Physiology, production and action of progesterone", *Acta Obstetricia et Gynecologica Scandinavica,* 2015; 94, pp.8–16

12 Reed, B.G., and Carr, B.R., "The normal menstrual cycle and the control of ovulation", *MDText.com, Inc.,* 5 August 2018. ncbi.nlm.nih.gov/books/NBK279054/

13 Barth, C., Villringer, A. and Sacher, J., "Sex hormones affect neurotransmitters and shape the adult female brain during hormonal transition periods", *Frontiers in Neuroscience,* 2015; 9

14 Scheuringer, A. and Pletzer, B., "Sex differences and menstrual cycle dependent changes in cognitive strategies during spatial navigation and verbal fluency", *Frontiers in Psychology,* 2017; 8

15 Hidalgo-Lopez, E. and Pletzer, B., "Interactive effects of dopamine baseline levels and cycle phase on executive functions: The role of progesterone", *Frontiers in Neuroscience,* 2017; 11

16 Sundström Poromaa, I. and Gingnell, M., "Menstrual cycle influence on cognitive function and emotion processing – from a reproductive perspective", *Frontiers in Neuroscience,* 2014; 8

17 Zierau, O., Zenclussen, A.C. and Jensen, F., "Role of female sex hormones, estradiol and progesterone, in mast cell behavior", *Frontiers in Immunology,* 2012; 3(169). ncbi.nlm.nih.gov/pmc/articles/PMC3377947/

18 Mlcek, J., Jurikova, T., Skrovankova, S. and Sochor, J., "Quercetin and its anti-allergic immune response", *Molecules,* 2016; 21(5), p.623. ncbi.nlm.nih.gov/pmc/articles/PMC6273625/

19 Takasaki, A., Tamura, H., Taniguchi, K., Asada, H., Taketani, T., Matsuoka, A., Yamagata, Y., Shimamura, K., Morioka, H. and Sugino, N., "Luteal blood flow and luteal function", *Journal of Ovarian Research,* 2009; 2(1), p.1

20 National Research Council (US) Committee on Diet and Health, "Fat-Soluble Vitamins", *Nih.gov*, 2016. ncbi.nlm.nih.gov/books/NBK218749/

21 US Department of Agriculture, Agriculture Research Service, *FoodData Central*, 2019. fdc.nal.usda.gov/index.html.

22 Kovacova-Hanuskova, E., Buday, T., Gavliakova, S. and Plevkova, J., "Histamine, histamine intoxication and intolerance", *Allergologia et Immunopathologia*, 2015; 43(5), pp.498–506

23 Randabunga, E.J., Lukas, E., Tumedia, J.L. and T. Chalid, S.M., "Effect of pyridoxine on prostaglandin plasma level for primary dysmenorrheal treatment", *Indonesian Journal of Obstetrics and Gynecology*, 2018; 6(4), Page #

24 Micronutrient Information Center, "Vitamin B6", Linus Pauling Institute, Oregon State University, 2019. lpi.oregonstate.edu/mic/vitamins/vitamin-B6

25 US Department of Agriculture, Agriculture Research Service, *FoodData Central*, 2019. fdc.nal.usda.gov/index.html.

26 Nair, R. and Maseeh, A., "Vitamin D: The 'sunshine' vitamin", *Journal of Pharmacology & Pharmacotherapeutics*, 2012; 3(2), pp.118–26. ncbi.nlm.nih.gov/pmc/articles/PMC3356951/

27 Łagowska, K., "The rationship between vitamin D status and the menstrual cycle in young women: A preliminary study", *Nutrients, Journal*, 2018; 10(11), p.1729

28 Dennis, N., Houghton, L., Pankhurst, M., Harper, M. and McLennan, I., "Acute supplementation with high dose vitamin D3 increases serum anti-müllerian hormone in young women", *Nutrients*, 2017; 9(7), p.719

29 Jukic, A.M.Z., Steiner, A.Z. and Baird, D.D., "Association between serum 25-hydroxyvitamin D and ovarian reserve in premenopausal women", *Menopause*, 2015; 22(3), pp.312–316

30 Moini, A., Ebrahimi, T., Shirzad, N., Hosseini, R., Radfar, M., Bandarian, F., Jafari-Adli, S., Qorbani, M. and Hemmatabadi, M., "The effect of vitamin D on primary dysmenorrhea with vitamin D deficiency: A randomized double-blind controlled clinical trial", *Gynecological Endocrinology*, 2016; 32(6), pp.502–505. pubmed.ncbi.nlm.nih.gov/27147120/

31 Pahwa, R., Goyal, A., Bansal, P. and Jialal, I., "Chronic Inflammation", *Statpearls*, 2019, ncbi.nlm.nih.gov/books/NBK493173/

32 Micronutrient Information Center, "Vitamin D", Linus Pauling Institute, Oregon State University, 2014. lpi.oregonstate.edu/mic/vitamins/vitamin-D

33 US Department of Agriculture, Agriculture Research Service, *FoodData Central*, 2019. fdc.nal.usda.gov/index.html.

34 Joseph, D. and Whirledge, S., "Stress and the HPA axis: Balancing homeostasis and fertility", *International Journal of Molecular Sciences*, 2017; 18(10), p.2224. ncbi.nlm.nih.gov/pmc/articles/PMC5666903/

35 Wohlgemuth, K.J., Arieta, L.R., Brewer, G.J., Hoselton, A.L., Gould, L.M. and Smith-Ryan, A.E., "Sex differences and considerations for female specific nutritional strategies: A narrative review", *Journal of the International Society of Sports Nutrition*, 2021; 18(1), Page #

Chapter 7

1 Brkić, M., "The role of E2/P ratio in the etiology of fibrocystic breast disease, mastalgia and mastodynia", *Acta Clinica Croatica*, 2018; 57(4), p.756

2 Kessler, J.H., "The effect of supraphysiologic levels of iodine on patients with cyclic mastalgia", *Breast Journal*, 2004; 10(4), pp.328–336

3 Murshid, K.R., "A review of mastalgia in patients with fibrocystic breast changes and the non-surgical treatment options", *Journal of Taibah University Medical Sciences*, 2011; 6(1), pp.1–18

4 De la Vieja, A. and Santisteban, P., "Role of iodide metabolism in physiology and cancer", *Endocrine-Related Cancer*, 2018; 25(4), pp.R225–R245

5 Gibson, D.A. and Saunders, P.T.K., "Endocrine disruption of oestrogen action and female reproductive tract cancers", *Endocrine-Related Cancer*, 2013; 21(2), pp.T13–T31

6 Street, M., Angelini, S., Bernasconi, S., Burgio, E., Cassio, A., Catellani, C., Cirillo, F., Deodati, A., Fabbrizi, E., Fanos, V., Gargano, G., Grossi, E., Iughetti, L., Lazzeroni, P., Mantovani, A., Migliore, L., Palanza, P., Panzica, G., Papini, A. and Parmigiani, S., "Current knowledge on endocrine disrupting chemicals (edcs) from animal biology to humans, from pregnancy to adulthood: Highlights from a national Italian meeting", *International Journal of Molecular Sciences*, 2018; 19(6), p.1647

7 D'Argenio, V., Dittfeld, L., Lazzeri, P., Tomaiuolo, R. and Tasciotti, E., "Unraveling the balance between genes, microbes, lifestyle and the environment to improve healthy reproduction", *Genes*, 2021; 12(4), p.605

8 National Institute of Environmental Health Sciences, "Endocrine disruptors", National Institute of Environmental Health Sciences, 2018. niehs.nih.gov/health/topics/agents/endocrine/index.cfm

9 Albini, A., Rosano, C., Angelini, G., Amaro, A., Esposito, A.I., Maramotti, S., Noonan, D.M. and Pfeffer, U., "Exogenous Hormonal regulation in breast cancer cells by phytoestrogens and endocrine disruptors", *Current Medicinal Chemistry*, 2014; 21, pp.1129–1145. ncbi.nlm.nih.gov/pmc/articles/PMC4153070/

10 Blackwell, L.F., Vigil, P., Cooke, D.G., d'Arcangues, C. and Brown, J.B., "Monitoring of ovarian activity by daily measurement of urinary excretion rates of oestrone glucuronide and pregnanediol glucuronide using the Ovarian Monitor, Part III: Variability of normal menstrual cycle profiles", *Human Reproduction*, 2013; 28(12), pp.3306–3315

11 Arendt, L.M. and Kuperwasser, C., "Form and function: How estrogen and progesterone regulate the mammary epithelial hierarchy", *Journal of Mammary Gland Biology and Neoplasia*, 2015; 20(1–2), pp.9–25

12 Raghunath, R.S., Venables, Z.C. and Millington, G.W.M., "The menstrual cycle and the skin", *Clinical and Experimental Dermatology*, 2015; 40(2), pp.111–115

13 Bull, J.R., Rowland, S.P., Scherwitzl, E.B., Scherwitzl, R., Danielsson, K.G. and Harper, J., "Real-world menstrual cycle characteristics of more than 600,000 menstrual cycles", *npj Digital Medicine*, 2019; 2(1), p.4

14 Vigil, P., Lyon, C., Flores, B., Rioseco, H. and Serrano, F., "Ovulation: A sign of health", *Linacre Quarterly*, 2017; 84(4), pp.343–355. ncbi.nlm.nih.gov/pmc/articles/PMC5730019/

15 Mesen, T.B. and Young, S.L., "Progesterone and the luteal phase", *Obstetrics and Gynecology Clinics of North America*, 2015; 42(1), pp.135–151

16 Rybaczyk, L.A., Bashaw, M.J., Pathak, D.R., Moody, S.M., Gilders, R.M. and Holzschu, D.L., "An overlooked connection: Serotonergic mediation of estrogen-related physiology and pathology", *BMC Women's Health*, 2005; 5(1). ncbi.nlm.nih.gov/pmc/articles/PMC1327664/

17 Manocha, M. and Khan, W.I., "Serotonin and GI disorders: An update on clinical and experimental studies", *Clinical and Translational Gastroenterology*, 2012;3(4), p.e13. ncbi.nlm.nih.gov/pmc/articles/PMC3365677/

18 Bistoletti, M., Bosi, A., Banfi, D., Giaroni, C. and Baj, A., "The microbiota-gut-brain axis: Focus on the fundamental communication pathways", *Progress in Molecular Biology and Translational Science*, 2020; 176, pp.43–110

19 Hamidovic, A., Karapetyan, K., Serdarevic, F., Choi, S.H., Eisenlohr-Moul, T. and Pinna, G., "Higher circulating cortisol in the follicular vs. luteal phase of the menstrual cycle: A meta-analysis", *Frontiers in Endocrinology*, 2020; 11

20 Holland, J., *Moody Bitches: The Truth about the Drugs You're Taking, the Sleep You're Missing, the Sex You're Not Having, and What's Really Making You Crazy*, Penguin Books, 2015, pp.36–40

21 American College of Obstetricians and Gynecologists, "ACOG PRACTICE BULLETIN", *International Journal of Gynecology & Obstetrics*, 2001; 73(2), pp.183–191

22 Draper, C.F., Duisters, K., Weger, B., Chakrabarti, A., Harms, A.C., Brennan, L., Hankemeier, T., Goulet, L., Konz, T., Martin, F.P., Moco, S. and van der Greef, J., "Menstrual cycle rhythmicity: Metabolic patterns in healthy women", *Scientific Reports*, 2018; 8. ncbi.nlm.nih.gov/pmc/articles/PMC6167362/

23 Rybaczyk, L.A., Bashaw, M.J., Pathak, D.R., Moody, S.M., Gilders, R.M. and Holzschu, D.L., "An overlooked connection: Serotonergic mediation

of estrogen-related physiology and pathology", *BMC Women's Health*, 2005; 5(1). ncbi.nlm.nih.gov/pmc/articles/PMC1327664/

24 Yabut, J.M., Crane, J.D., Green, A.E., Keating, D.J., Khan, W.I. and Steinberg, G.R., "Emerging roles for serotonin in regulating metabolism: New implications for an ancient molecule", *Endocrine Reviews*, 2019; 40(4), pp.1092–1107. academic.oup.com/edrv/article/40/4/1092/5406261

25 Draper, C.F., Duisters, K., Weger, B., Chakrabarti, A., Harms, A.C., Brennan, L., Hankemeier, T., Goulet, L., Konz, T., Martin, F.P., Moco, S. and van der Greef, J., "Menstrual cycle rhythmicity: Metabolic patterns in healthy women", *Scientific Reports*, 2018; 8. ncbi.nlm.nih.gov/pmc/articles/PMC6167362/

26 Ibid.

27 Wohlgemuth, K.J., Arieta, L.R., Brewer, G.J., Hoselton, A.L., Gould, L.M. and Smith-Ryan, A.E., "Sex differences and considerations for female specific nutritional strategies: A narrative review", *Journal of the International Society of Sports Nutrition*, 2021; 18(1), p.3

28 Henmi, H., Endo, T., Kitajima, Y., Manase, K., Hata, H. and Kudo, R., "Effects of ascorbic acid supplementation on serum progesterone levels in patients with a luteal phase defect", *Fertility and Sterility*, 2003; 80(2), pp.459–461

29 Takasaki, A., Tamura, H., Taniguchi, K., Asada, H., Taketani, T., Matsuoka, A., Yamagata, Y., Shimamura, K., Morioka, H. and Sugino, N., "Luteal blood flow and luteal function", *Journal of Ovarian Research*, 2009; 2(1), p.1

30 US Department of Agriculture, Agriculture Research Service, *FoodData Central*, 2019. fdc.nal.usda.gov/index.html.

31 Hodges, J., Cao, S., Cladis, D. and Weaver, C., "Lactose intolerance and bone health: The challenge of ensuring adequate calcium intake", *Nutrients*, 2019; 11(4), p.718

32 Ibid.

33 Abdi, F., Ozgoli, G. and Rahnemaie, F.S., "A systematic review of the role of vitamin D and calcium in premenstrual syndrome", *Obstetrics & Gynecology Science*, 2019; 62(2), p.73

34 Lanje, M.A., Bhutey, A.K., Kulkarni, S.R., Dhawle, U.P. and Sande, A.S., "Serum electrolytes during different phases of menstrual cycle", *International Journal of Pharma Sciences and Research*, 2010; 1(10), pp.435–437. researchgate.net/publication/50434417_Serum_Electrolytes_During_Different_Phases_Of_Menstrual_Cycle

35 Micronutrient Information Center, "Calcium", Linus Pauling Institute, Oregon State University, 2014. lpi.oregonstate.edu/mic/minerals/calcium

36 US Department of Agriculture, Agriculture Research Service, *FoodData Central*, 2019. fdc.nal.usda.gov/index.html.

37 Office of Dietary Supplements, "Potassium", *National Institutes of Health*, 2016. ods.od.nih.gov/factsheets/Potassium-HealthProfessional/

38 Chocano-Bedoya, P.O., Manson, J.E., Hankinson, S.E., Johnson, S.R., Chasan-Taber, L., Ronnenberg, A.G., Bigelow, C. and Bertone-

Johnson, E.R., "Intake of selected minerals and risk of premenstrual syndrome", *American Journal of Epidemiology*, 2013; 177(10), pp.1118–1127. ncbi.nlm.nih.gov/pmc/articles/PMC3649635/

39 Lanje, M.A., Bhutey, A.K., Kulkarni, S.R., Dhawle, U.P. and Sande, A.S., "Serum electrolytes during different phases of menstrual cycle", *International Journal of Pharma Sciences and Research*, 2010; 1(10), pp.435–437. researchgate.net/publication/50434417_Serum_Electrolytes_During_Different_Phases_Of_Menstrual_Cycle

40 US Department of Agriculture, Agriculture Research Service, *FoodData Central*, 2019. fdc.nal.usda.gov/index.html.

41 British Dietetic Association, "Salt", BDA, 2010. bda.uk.com/resource/salt.html

42 Krela-Kaźmierczak, I., Czarnywojtek, A., Skoracka, K., Rychter, A.M., Ratajczak, A.E., Szymczak-Tomczak, A., Ruchała, M. and Dobrowolska, A., "Is there an ideal diet to protect against iodine deficiency?", *PubMed.gov*, 2021; 13(2), p.513. pubmed.ncbi.nlm.nih.gov/33557336/

43 Santos, J.A.R., Christoforou, A., Trieu, K., McKenzie, B.L., Downs, S., Billot, L., Webster, J. and Li, M., "Iodine fortification of foods and condiments, other than salt, for preventing iodine deficiency disorders", *Cochrane Database of Systematic Reviews*, 2019; 2(2), p.9

44 British Dietetics Association, "Iodine Food fact Sheet", BDA, 2019. bda.uk.com/resource/iodine.html

45 US Department of Agriculture, Agriculture Research Service, *FoodData Central*, 2019. fdc.nal.usda.gov/index.html.

46 Lovallo, W.R., Whitsett, T.L., al'Absi, M., Sung, B.H., Vincent, A.S. and Wilson, M.F., "Caffeine stimulation of cortisol secretion across the waking hours in relation to caffeine intake levels", *Psychosomatic medicine*, 2005; 67(5), pp.734–9. ncbi.nlm.nih.gov/pubmed/16204431

Chapter 8

1 Latthe, P., Champaneria, R. and Khan, K., "Dysmenorrhea", *American Family Physician*, 2012; 85(4), pp.386–387. aafp.org/afp/2012/0215/p386.html

2 Schoep, M.E., Adang, E.M.M., Maas, J.W.M., De Bie, B., Aarts, J.W.M. and Nieboer, T.E., "Productivity loss due to menstruation-related symptoms: A nationwide cross-sectional survey among 32 748 women", *BMJ Open*, 2019; 9(6), p.e026186

3 The Libresse Pain Project, 2021. libresse-images.essity.com/images-c5/699/322699/original/pain-report-final-pdf.pdf

4 Munro, M.G., Critchley, H.O.D. and Fraser, I.S., "The two FIGO systems for normal and abnormal uterine bleeding symptoms and classification of causes of abnormal uterine bleeding in the reproductive years: 2018 revisions", *International Journal of Gynecology & Obstetrics*, 2018; 143(3), pp.393–408

5   Raja, S.N., Carr, D.B., Cohen, M., Finnerup, N.B., Flor, H., Gibson, S., Keefe, F.J., Mogil, J.S., Ringkamp, M., Sluka, K.A., Song, X.-J., Stevens, B., Sullivan, M.D., Tutelman, P.R., Ushida, T. and Vader, K., "The revised International Association for the Study of Pain definition of pain: Concepts, challenges, and compromises", *PAIN*, 2020; 161(9), pp.1976–1982. journals.lww. com/pain/Abstract/9000/The_revised_International_Association_for_ the.98346.aspx

6   Ricciotti, E. and FitzGerald, G.A., "Prostaglandins and inflammation", *Arteriosclerosis, Thrombosis, and Vascular Biology*, 2011; 31(5), pp.986–1000.

7   Pahwa, R., Goyal, A., Bansal, P. and Jialal, I., "Chronic Inflammation", *Statpearls*, 2019, ncbi.nlm.nih.gov/books/NBK493173/

8   World Health Organization, *The top 10 causes of death*, 2010. who.int/ news-room/fact-sheets/detail/the-top-10-causes-of-death

9   Pahwa, R., Goyal, A., Bansal, P. and Jialal, I., "Chronic Inflammation", *Statpearls*, 2019, ncbi.nlm.nih.gov/books/NBK493173/

10 Gold, E.B., Wells, C. and Rasor, M.O., "The association of inflammation with premenstrual symptoms", *Journal of Women's Health*, 2016; 25(9), pp.865–874

11 Proctor, M. and Farquhar, C., "Diagnosis and management of dysmenorrhoea", *BMJ*, 2006; 332(7550), pp.1134–1138. ncbi.nlm.nih.gov/ pmc/articles/PMC1459624/

12 Smith, R.P., *Dysmenorrhea and Menorrhagia: A Clinician's Guide*, Springer, 2019, pp.84–85

13 Barcikowska, Z., Rajkowska-Labon, E., Grzybowska, M.E., Hansdorfer-Korzon, R. and Zorena, K., "Inflammatory markers in dysmenorrhea and therapeutic options", *International Journal of Environmental Research and Public Health*, 2020; 17(4). ncbi.nlm.nih.gov/pmc/articles/ PMC7068519/

14 Ibid.

15 Hoyle, A.T. and Puckett, Y., "Endometrioma", *PubMed*, 2021. ncbi.nlm.nih. gov/books/NBK559230/

16 Porpora, M.G., Brunelli, R., Costa, G., Imperiale, L., Krasnowska, E.K., Lundeberg, T., Nofroni, I., Piccioni, M.G., Pittaluga, E., Ticino, A. and Parasassi, T., "A promise in the treatment of endometriosis: An observational cohort study on ovarian endometrioma reduction by n-acetylcysteine", *Evidence-based Complementary and Alternative Medicine*, 2013. ncbi.nlm.nih.gov/pmc/articles/PMC3662115/

17 Teimoori, B., Ghasemi, M., Sadat Amir Hoseini, Z. and Razavi, M., "The efficacy of zinc administration in the treatment of primary dysmenorrhea", *Oman Medical Journal*, 2016; 31(2), pp.107–111

18 Edwards, S.E., Rocha, I., Williamson, E.M. and Heinrich, M., *Phytopharmacy: An Evidence-based Guide to Herbal Medicinal Products*. Wiley Blackwell, 2015, pp.118–119

19 Vučković, S., Srebro, D., Vujović, K.S., Vučetić, Č. and Prostran, M., "Cannabinoids and pain: New insights from old molecules", *Frontiers in Pharmacology*, 2018, 9. frontiersin.org/articles/10.3389/fphar.2018.01259/full

20 Klein, T.W., "Cannabinoid-based drugs as anti-inflammatory therapeutics", *Nature Reviews Immunology*, 2005; 5(5), pp.400–411

21 Proctor, M., Farquhar, C., Stones, W., He, L., Zhu, X. and Brown, J., "Transcutaneous electrical nerve stimulation for primary dysmenorrhoea", *Cochrane Database of Systematic Reviews*, 2002, p.12

22 Akin, M., "Continuous low-level topical heat in the treatment of dysmenorrhea", *Obstetrics & Gynecology*, 2001; 97(3), pp.343–349

23 Jo, J. and Lee, S.H., "Heat therapy for primary dysmenorrhea: A systematic review and meta-analysis of its effects on pain relief and quality of life", *Scientific Reports*, 2018; 8(1)

24 Rogers, P.A.W., D'Hooghe, T.M., Fazleabas, A., Gargett, C.E., Giudice, L.C., Montgomery, G.W., Rombauts, L., Salamonsen, L.A. and Zondervan, K.T., "Priorities for endometriosis research: Recommendations from an international consensus workshop", *Reproductive Sciences*, 2009; 16(4), pp.335–346

25 Agarwal, S.K., Chapron, C., Giudice, L.C., Laufer, M.R., Leyland, N., Missmer, S.A., Singh, S.S. and Taylor, H.S., "Clinical diagnosis of endometriosis: A call to action", *American Journal of Obstetrics and Gynecology*, 2019; 220(4), pp.354.e1–354.e12. sciencedirect.com/science/article/pii/S000293781930002X

26 Morassutto, C., Monasta, L., Ricci, G., Barbone, F. and Ronfani, L., "Incidence and estimated prevalence of endometriosis and adenomyosis in northeast Italy: A data linkage study", *PLOS One*, 2016; 11(4), p.e0154227

27 Hudelist, G., Fritzer, N., Thomas, A., Niehues, C., Oppelt, P., Haas, D., Tammaa, A. and Salzer, H., "Diagnostic delay for endometriosis in Austria and Germany: Causes and possible consequences", *Human Reproduction*, 2012; 27(12), pp.3412–3416

28 Vercellini, P., Viganò, P., Somigliana, E. and Fedele, L., "Endometriosis: Pathogenesis and treatment", *Nature Reviews Endocrinology*, 2013; 10(5), pp.261–275

29 American Society For Reproductive Medicine, "Endometriosis: A guide for patients", *Patient Information Series*, 2016. reproductivefacts.org/globalassets/rf/news-and-publications/bookletsfact-sheets/english-fact-sheets-and-info-booklets/booklet_endometriosis.pdf

30 Mueller, A., Siemer, J., Schreiner, S., Koesztner, H., Hoffmann, I., Binder, H., Beckmann, M.W. and Dittrich, R., "Role of estrogen and progesterone in the regulation of uterine peristalsis: Results from perfused non-pregnant swine uteri", *Human Reproduction*, 2006; 21(7), pp.1863–1868

31 Ham, E.A., Cirillo, V.J., Zanetti, M.E. and Kuehl, F.A., "Estrogen-directed synthesis of specific prostaglandins in uterus", *Proceedings of the National Academy of Sciences*, 1975; 72(4), pp.1420–1424

32 Crinnion, W.J., "Toxic effects of the easily avoidable phthalates and parabens", *Alternative Medicine Review: A Journal of Clinical Therapeutic*, 2010; 15(3), pp.190–196. pubmed.ncbi.nlm.nih.gov/21155623/

33 Samavat, H. and Kurzer, M.S., "Estrogen metabolism and breast cancer", *Cancer Letters*, 2015; 356(2), pp.231–243. ncbi.nlm.nih.gov/pmc/articles/PMC4505810/

34 Hodges, R.E. and Minich, D.M., "Modulation of metabolic detoxification pathways using foods and food-derived components: A scientific review with clinical application", *Journal of Nutrition and Metabolism*, 2015, pp.1–23

35 De Figueiredo, S., Binda, N., Nogueira-Machado, J., Vieira-Filho, S. and Caligiorne, R., "The antioxidant properties of organosulfur compounds (sulforaphane)", *Recent Patents on Endocrine, Metabolic & Immune Drug Discovery*, 2015; 9(1), pp.24–39

36 Hodges, R.E. and Minich, D.M., "Modulation of metabolic detoxification pathways using foods and food-derived components: A scientific review with clinical application", *Journal of Nutrition and Metabolism*, 2015, pp.1–23

37 De Figueiredo, S., Binda, N., Nogueira-Machado, J., Vieira-Filho, S. and Caligiorne, R., "The antioxidant properties of organosulfur compounds (sulforaphane)", *Recent Patents on Endocrine, Metabolic & Immune Drug Discovery*, 21015; 9(1), pp.24–39

38 Plottel, C.S. and Blaser, M.J., "Microbiome and malignancy", *Cell Host & Microbe*, 2011; 10(4), pp.324–335

39 Ibid.

40 Hodges, R.E. and Minich, D.M., "Modulation of metabolic detoxification pathways using foods and food-derived components: A scientific review with clinical application", *Journal of Nutrition and Metabolism*, 2015, pp.1–23

41 Kwa, M., S. Plottel, C., J. Blaser, M. and Adams, S., "The intestinal microbiome and estrogen receptor–positive female breast cancer", *Journal of the National Cancer Institute*, 2016; 108(8), p.2

42 Maruti, S.S., Li, L., Chang, J.-L., Prunty, J., Schwarz, Y., Li, S.S., King, I.B., Potter, J.D. and Lampe, J.W., "Dietary and demographic correlates of serum ß-glucuronidase activity", *Nutrition and Cancer*, 2010; 62(2), pp.208–219

43 Hutkins, R.W., Krumbeck, J.A., Bindels, L.B., Cani, P.D., Fahey, G., Goh, Y.J., Hamaker, B., Martens, E.C., Mills, D.A., Rastal, R.A., Vaughan, E. and Sanders, M.E., "Prebiotics: Why definitions matter", *Current Opinion in Biotechnology*, 2016; 37(37), pp.1–7

44 Rezac, S., Kok, C.R., Heermann, M. and Hutkins, R., "Fermented foods as a dietary source of live organisms", *Frontiers in Microbiology*, 2018; 9. ncbi.nlm.nih.gov/pmc/articles/PMC6117398/

45 De Preter, V., Raemen, H., Cloetens, L., Houben, E., Rutgeerts, P. and Verbeke, K., "Effect of dietary intervention with different pre- and probiotics on intestinal bacterial enzyme activities", *European Journal of Clinical Nutrition*, 2007; 62(2), pp.225–231

46 Drăghici, I.M., Drăghici, L., Cojocaru, M., Gorgan, C.L. and Vrabie, C.D., "The immunoprofile of interstitial Cajal cells within adenomyosis/endometriosis lesions", *Romanian Journal of Morphology and Embryology*, 2015; 56(1), pp.133–138

47 guysandstthomas.nhs.uk/resources/patient-information/gynaecology/adenomyosis.pdf

48 Krentel, H., Cezar, C., Becker, S., Di Spiezio Sardo, A., Tanos, V., Wallwiener, M. and De Wilde, R.L., "From clinical symptoms to MR imaging: Diagnostic steps in adenomyosis", *BioMed Research International*, 2017, pp.1–6

49 Vannuccini, S. and Petraglia, F., "Recent advances in understanding and managing adenomyosis", *F1000Research*, 2019; 8(8), p.283

50 guysandstthomas.nhs.uk/resources/patient-information/gynaecology/Fibroids.pdf

51 Ibid.

52 Eltoukhi, H.M., Modi, M.N., Weston, M., Armstrong, A.Y. and Stewart, E.A., "The health disparities of uterine fibroid tumors for African American women: A public health issue", *American Journal of Obstetrics and Gynecology*, 2014; 210(3), pp.194–199

53 Ibid.

54 Baird, D.D., Dunson, D.B., Hill, M.C., Cousins, D. and Schectman, J.M., "High cumulative incidence of uterine leiomyoma in black and white women: Ultrasound evidence", *American Journal of Obstetrics and Gynecology*, 2003; 188(1), pp.100–107

55 Baird, D.D., Hill, M.C., Schectman, J.M. and Hollis, B.W., "Vitamin D and the risk of uterine fibroids", *Epidemiology*, 2013; 24(3), pp.447–453

56 Eltoukhi, H.M., Modi, M.N., Weston, M., Armstrong, A.Y. and Stewart, E.A., "The health disparities of uterine fibroid tumors for African American women: A public health issue", *American Journal of Obstetrics and Gynecology*, 2014; 210(3), pp.194–199

57 NHS, "Ovarian cyst", 2017. nhs.uk/conditions/ovarian-cyst/

58 Institute for Quality and Efficiency in Health Care, "Ovarian cysts: Overview", *InformedHealth.org*, 2019. ncbi.nlm.nih.gov/books/NBK539572/

Chapter 9

1   Cowen, A.S. and Keltner, D., "Self-report captures 27 distinct categories of emotion bridged by continuous gradients", *Proceedings of the National Academy of Sciences*, 2017; 114(38), pp.E7900–E7909. pnas.org/content/114/38/E7900

2   Holland, J., *Moody Bitches: The Truth about the Drugs You're Taking, the Sleep You're Missing, the Sex You're Not Having, and What's Really Making You Crazy*, Penguin Books, 2015, pp.36–40

3   Mishra, S. and Marwaha, R., "Premenstrual Dysphoric Disorder", *StatPearls*, 2018. ncbi.nlm.nih.gov/books/NBK532307/

4   Wittchen, H.-U., Perkonigg, A. and Pfister, H., "Trauma and PTSD? An overlooked pathogenic pathway for premenstrual dysphoric disorder?", *Archives of Women's Mental Health*, 2013; 6(4), pp.293–297

5   Dubey, N., Hoffman, J.F., Schuebel, K., Yuan, Q., Martinez, P.E., Nieman, L.K., Rubinow, D.R., Schmidt, P.J. and Goldman, D., "The ESC/E(Z) complex, an effector of response to ovarian steroids, manifests an intrinsic difference in cells from women with premenstrual dysphoric disorder", *Molecular Psychiatry*, 2017; 22(8), pp.1172–1184

6   Straneva, P.A., Maixner, W., Light, K.C., Pedersen, C.A., Costello, N.L. and Girdler, S.S., "Menstrual cycle, beta-endorphins, and pain sensitivity in premenstrual dysphoric disorder", *Health Psychology*, 2002; 21(4), pp.358–367

7   Hantsoo, L. and Epperson, C.N., "Allopregnanolone in premenstrual dysphoric disorder (PMDD): Evidence for dysregulated sensitivity to GABA-A receptor modulating neuroactive steroids across the menstrual cycle", *Neurobiology of Stress*, 2020; 12. sciencedirect.com/science/article/pii/S2352289520300035

8   Hartlage, S.A., "Criteria for premenstrual dysphoric disorder", *Archives of General Psychiatry*, 2012; 69(3), p.300. jamanetwork.com/journals/jamapsychiatry/fullarticle/1107411

9   Reid, R.L., "Table 1: Diagnostic criteria for premenstrual dysphoric disorder (PMDD), *Endotext.org*, 2017. ncbi.nlm.nih.gov/books/NBK279045/table/premenstrual-syndrom.table1diag/

10 Epperson, C.N., Steiner, M., Hartlage, S.A., Eriksson, E., Schmidt, P.J., Jones, I. and Yonkers, K.A., "Premenstrual dysphoric disorder: Evidence for a new category for DSM-5" *American Journal of Psychiatry*, 2012; 169(5), pp.465–475

11 Retallick-Brown, H., Blampied, N. and Rucklidge, J.J., "A pilot randomized treatment-controlled trial comparing vitamin B6 with broad-spectrum micronutrients for premenstrual syndrome", *Journal of Alternative and Complementary Medicine*, 2020; 26(2), pp.88–97.

12 Kennedy, D., "B vitamins and the brain: Mechanisms, dose and efficacy – a review", *Nutrients*, 2016; 8(2), p.68. ncbi.nlm.nih.gov/pmc/articles/PMC4772032/

13 Weise, C., Kaiser, G., Janda, C., Kues, Johanna N., Andersson, G., Strahler, J. and Kleinstäuber, M., "Internet-based cognitive-behavioural intervention for women with premenstrual dysphoric disorder: A randomized controlled trial", *Psychotherapy and Psychosomatics*, 2019; 88(1), pp.16–29

14 Hantsoo, L. and Epperson, C.N., "Premenstrual dysphoric disorder: Epidemiology and treatment", *Current Psychiatry Reports*, 2015; 17(11). ncbi.nlm.nih.gov/pmc/articles/PMC4890701/

15 Spring, B., "Recent research on the behavioral effects of tryptophan and carbohydrate", *Nutrition and Health*, 1984; 3(1–2), pp.55–67

16 Csikszentmihalyi, M., *Flow: The Psychology of Optimal Experience*, Harper & Row, 1990

17 Schmidt, P.J., Nieman, L.K., Danaceau, M.A., Adams, L.F. and Rubinow, D.R., "Differential behavioral effects of gonadal steroids in women with and in those without premenstrual syndrome", *New England Journal of Medicine*, 1998; 338(4), pp.209–216

18 Rapkin, A.J. and Akopians, A.L., "Pathophysiology of premenstrual syndrome and premenstrual dysphoric disorder", *Menopause International*, 2012; 18(2), pp.52–9. ncbi.nlm.nih.gov/pubmed/22611222

19 Bu, L., Lai, Y., Deng, Y., Xiong, C., Li, F., Li, L., Suzuki, K., Ma, S. and Liu, C., "Negative mood is associated with diet and dietary antioxidants in university students during the menstrual cycle: A cross-sectional study from Guangzhou, China", *Antioxidants*, 2019; 9(1), p.23

20 Haam, J. and Yakel, J.L., "Cholinergic modulation of the hippocampal region and memory function", *Journal of Neurochemistry*, 2017; 142(S2), pp.111–121

21 Juárez Olguín, H., Calderón Guzmán, D., Hernández García, E. and Barragán Mejía, G., "The role of dopamine and its dysfunction as a consequence of oxidative stress", *Oxidative Medicine and Cellular Longevity*, 2016, pp.1–13. hindawi.com/journals/omcl/2016/9730467/

22 Berger, M., Gray, J.A. and Roth, B.L., "The expanded biology of serotonin", *Annual Review of Medicine*, 2009; 60, pp.355–66. ncbi.nlm.nih.gov/pubmed/19630576

23 Jewett, B.E. and Sharma, S., "Physiology, GABA", *StatPearls*, 2020. ncbi.nlm.nih.gov/books/NBK513311/

24 Kroese, F.M., De Ridder, D.T.D., Evers, C. and Adriaanse, M.A., "Bedtime procrastination: Introducing a new area of procrastination", *Frontiers in Psychology*, 2014; 5(611). ncbi.nlm.nih.gov/pmc/articles/PMC4062817/

25 Kamphorst, B.A., Nauts, S., De Ridder, D.T.D. and Anderson, J.H., "Too depleted to turn in: The relevance of end-of-the-day resource depletion for reducing bedtime procrastination", *Frontiers in Psychology*, 2018; 9(252), p.1

26 Basso, J.C. and Suzuki, W.A., "The effects of acute exercise on mood, cognition, neurophysiology, and neurochemical pathways: A

review", *Brain Plasticity*, 2017; 2(2), pp.127–152. content.iospress.com/articles/brain-plasticity/bpl160040

27 Strandwitz, P., "Neurotransmitter modulation by the gut microbiota", *Brain Research*, 2018; 1693(B), pp.128–133. ncbi.nlm.nih.gov/pubmed/29903615

28 Wang, H., Braun, C., Murphy, E.F. and Enck, P., "Bifidobacterium longum 1714™ strain modulates brain activity of healthy volunteers during social stress", *American Journal of Gastroenterology*, 2019; 114(7), pp.1152–1162. journals.lww.com/ajg/pages/articleviewer.aspx?year=2019&issue=07000&article=00025&type=Fulltext

29 Chaiyasut, C. and Sundaram Sivamaruthi, B., "Influence of probiotic supplementation on brain function: Involvement of gut microbiome, inflammation, and stress pathway", *Gut Microbiota – Brain Axis*, 2018

30 Messaoudi, M., Violle, N., Bisson, J.-F., Desor, D., Javelot, H. and Rougeot, C., "Beneficial psychological effects of a probiotic formulation (Lactobacillus helveticusR0052 and Bifidobacterium longumR0175) in healthy human volunteers", *Gut Microbes*, 2011; 2(4), pp.256–261

31 Kato-Kataoka, A., Nishida, K., Takada, M., Kawai, M., Kikuchi-Hayakawa, H., Suda, K., Ishikawa, H., Gondo, Y., Shimizu, K., Matsuki, T., Kushiro, A., Hoshi, R., Watanabe, O., Igarashi, T., Miyazaki, K., Kuwano, Y. and Rokutan, K., "Fermented milk containing lactobacillus casei strain shirota preserves the diversity of the gut microbiota and relieves abdominal dysfunction in healthy medical students exposed to academic stress", *Applied and Environmental Microbiology*, 2016; 82(12), pp.3649–3658. ncbi.nlm.nih.gov/pmc/articles/PMC4959178/

32 Reis, D.J., Ilardi, S.S. and Punt, S.E.W., "The anxiolytic effect of probiotics: A systematic review and meta-analysis of the clinical and preclinical literature", *PLOS One*, 2018; 13(6), p.e0199041

33 Hidese, S., Ogawa, S., Ota, M., Ishida, I., Yasukawa, Z., Ozeki, M. and Kunugi, H., "Effects of L-theanine administration on stress-related symptoms and cognitive functions in healthy adults: A randomized controlled trial", *Nutrients*, 2019; 11(10), p.2362

34 Sansone, R.A. and Sansone, L.A., "Sunshine, serotonin, and skin: A partial explanation for seasonal patterns in psychopathology?", *Innovations in Clinical Neuroscience*, 2013; 10(7-8), pp.20–24. ncbi.nlm.nih.gov/pmc/articles/PMC3779905/

35 Harrison, S.J., Tyrer, A.E., Levitan, R.D., Xu, X., Houle, S., Wilson, A.A., Nobrega, J.N., Rusjan, P.M. and Meyer, J.H., "Light therapy and serotonin transporter binding in the anterior cingulate and prefrontal cortex", *Acta Psychiatrica Scandinavica*, 2015; 132(5), pp.379–388

36 Weil, A., "Three breathing exercises and techniques", *Andrew Weil, MD*, 2019. drweil.com/health-wellness/body-mind-spirit/stress-anxiety/breathing-three-exercises/

Chapter 10

1 NHS Choices, "Polycystic ovary syndrome", 2019. nhs.uk/conditions/
   polycystic-ovary-syndrome-pcos/

2 Patel, S., "Polycystic ovary syndrome (PCOS): An inflammatory, systemic,
   lifestyle endocrinopathy", *Journal of Steroid Biochemistry and Molecular
   Biology*, 2018; 182, pp.27–36. sciencedirect.com/science/article/pii/
   S0960076018300396

3 NHS Choices, "Polycystic ovary syndrome", 2019. nhs.uk/conditions/
   polycystic-ovary-syndrome-pcos/

4 Goodarzi, M.O., Dumesic, D.A., Chazenbalk, G. and Azziz, R., "Polycystic
   ovary syndrome: Etiology, pathogenesis and diagnosis", *Nature
   Reviews Endocrinology*, 2011; 7(4), pp.219–231. nature.com/articles/
   nrendo.2010.217

5 Lizneva, D., Suturina, L., Walker, W., Brakta, S., Gavrilova-Jordan, L. and
   Azziz, R., "Criteria, prevalence, and phenotypes of polycystic ovary
   syndrome", *Fertility and Sterility*, 2016; 106(1), pp.6–15. sciencedirect.com/
   science/article/pii/S0015028216612323

6 Cheung, A.P. and Cog, F.,. "Polycystic ovary syndrome: A contemporary
   view", *Journal of Obstetrics and Gynaecology Canada*, 2010; 32(5),
   pp.423–425

7 Goodarzi, M.O., Dumesic, D.A., Chazenbalk, G. and Azziz, R., "Polycystic
   ovary syndrome: Etiology, pathogenesis and diagnosis", *Nature
   Reviews Endocrinology*, 2011; 7(4), pp.219–231. nature.com/articles/
   nrendo.2010.217

8 Lizneva, D., Suturina, L., Walker, W., Brakta, S., Gavrilova-Jordan, L. and
   Azziz, R., "Criteria, prevalence, and phenotypes of polycystic ovary
   syndrome", *Fertility and Sterility*, 2016; 106(1), pp.6–15. sciencedirect.com/
   science/article/pii/S0015028216612323

9 Hamilton-Fairley, D. and Taylor, A., "Anovulation", *BMJ*, 2003; 327(7414),
   pp.546–549

10 Delcour, C., Robin, G., Young, J. and Dewailly, D., "PCOS and
   hyperprolactinemia: What do we know in 2019?", *Clinical Medicine
   Insights: Reproductive Health*, 2019, 13, p.117955811987192

11 Goodarzi, M.O., Dumesic, D.A., Chazenbalk, G. and Azziz, R., "Polycystic
   ovary syndrome: Etiology, pathogenesis and diagnosis", *Nature
   Reviews Endocrinology*, 2011; 7(4), pp.219–231. nature.com/articles/
   nrendo.2010.217

12 Ibid.

13 Rodriguez Paris, V. and Bertoldo, M.J., "The mechanism of androgen
   actions in PCOS etiology", *Medical Sciences*, 2019; 7(9). ncbi.nlm.nih.gov/
   pmc/articles/PMC6780983/

14 Melnik, B.C. and Schmitz, G., "Role of insulin, insulin-like growth factor-1,
   hyperglycaemic food and milk consumption in the pathogenesis of acne
   vulgaris", *Experimental Dermatology*, 2009; 18(10), pp.833–841

15 Thomson, C.A., Ho, E. and Strom, M.B., "Chemopreventive properties of 3,3'-diindolylmethane in breast cancer: Evidence from experimental and human studies", *Nutrition Reviews*, 2016; 74(7), pp.432–443. ncbi.nlm.nih. gov/pmc/articles/PMC5059820/

16 Hwang, C., Sethi, S., Heilbrun, L.K., Gupta, N.S., Chitale, D.A., Sakr, W.A., Menon, M., Peabody, J.O., Smith, D.W., Sarkar, F.H. and Heath, E.I., "Anti-androgenic activity of absorption-enhanced 3, 3'-diindolylmethane in prostatectomy patients", *American Journal of Translational Research*, 2006; 8(1), pp.166–176. ncbi.nlm.nih.gov/pmc/articles/PMC4759426/. Accessed 10 Aug. 2021

17 Akdoğan, M., Tamer, M.N., Cüre, E., Cüre, M.C., Köroğlu, B.K. and Delibaş, N., "Effect of spearmint (Mentha spicata Labiatae) teas on androgen levels in women with hirsutism", *Phytotherapy Research: PTR*, 2007; 21(5), pp.444–447. ncbi.nlm.nih.gov/pubmed/17310494. Accessed 17 Aug. 2019

18 Grant, P. and Ramasamy, S., "An update on plant derived anti-androgens", *International Journal of Endocrinology and Metabolism*, 2012; 10(2), pp.497–502. ncbi.nlm.nih.gov/pmc/articles/PMC3693613/

19 Kogure, G.S., Miranda-Furtado, C.L., Silva, R.C., Melo, A.S., Ferriani, R.A., De Sá, M.F.S. and Reis, R.M.D., "Resistance exercise impacts lean muscle mass in women with polycystic ovary syndrome", *Medicine & Science in Sports & Exercise*, 2016; 48(4), pp.589–598. journals.lww.com/acsm-msse/Fulltext/2016/04000/Resistance_Exercise_Impacts_Lean_Muscle_Mass_in.2.aspx. Accessed 6 Jun. 2020

20 Nasiadek, M., Stragierowicz, J., Klimczak, M. and Kilanowicz, A., "The role of zinc in selected female reproductive system disorders", *Nutrients*, 2020; 12(8), p.2464

21 Goodarzi, M.O., "Looking for polycystic ovary syndrome genes: Rational and best strategy", *Seminars in Reproductive Medicine*, 2008; 26(1), pp.5–13

22 McRae, M.P., "Dietary fiber intake and type 2 diabetes mellitus: An umbrella review of meta-analyses", *Journal of Chiropractic Medicine*, 2018; 17(1), pp.44–53

23 Haidari, F., Banaei-Jahromi, N., Zakerkish, M. and Ahmadi, K., "The effects of flaxseed supplementation on metabolic status in women with polycystic ovary syndrome: A randomized open-labeled controlled clinical trial", *Nutrition Journal*, 2020; 19(1), p.5

24 Knowler, W.C., Barrett-Connor, E., Fowler, S.E., Hamman, R.F., Lachin, J.M., Walker, E.A. and Nathan, D.M., "Reduction in the incidence of type 2 diabetes with lifestyle intervention or metformin", *New England Journal of Medicine*, 2002; 346(6), pp.393–403. ncbi.nlm.nih.gov/pubmed/11832527

25 Santos, I.K. dos, Nunes, F.A.S. de S., Queiros, V.S., Cobucci, R.N., Dantas, P.B., Soares, G.M., Cabral, B.G. de A.T., Maranhão, T.M. de O. and Dantas, P.M.S., "Effect of high-intensity interval training on metabolic parameters

in women with polycystic ovary syndrome: A systematic review and meta-analysis of randomized controlled trials", *PLOS One*, 2021; 16(1), p.e0245023

26 Miranda-Furtado, C.L., Ramos, F.K.P., Kogure, G.S., Santana-Lemos, B.A., Ferriani, R.A., Calado, R.T. and dos Reis, R.M., "A nonrandomized trial of progressive resistance training intervention in women with polycystic ovary syndrome and its implications in telomere content", *Reproductive Sciences*, 2015; 23(5), pp.644–654

27 Ozay, A.C., Emekci Ozay, O., Okyay, R.E., Cagliyan, E., Kume, T. and Gulekli, B., "Different effects of myoinositol plus folic acid versus combined oral treatment on androgen levels in PCOS women", *International Journal of Endocrinology*, 2016, pp.1–8

28 González, F., "Inflammation in polycystic ovary syndrome: Underpinning of insulin resistance and ovarian dysfunction", *Steroids*, 2012; 77(4), pp.300–305

29 Minich, D.M. and Brown, B.I., "A review of dietary (phyto)nutrients for glutathione support", *Nutrients*, 2019; 11(9), p.2073

30 Mullington, J.M., Simpson, N.S., Meier-Ewert, H.K. and Haack, M., "Sleep loss and inflammation", *Best Practice & Research Clinical Endocrinology & Metabolism*, 2010; 24(5), pp.775–784. ncbi.nlm.nih.gov/pmc/articles/PMC3548567/

31 Jung, C.M., Khalsa, S.B.S., Scheer, F.A.J.L., Cajochen, C., Lockley, S.W., Czeisler, C.A. and Wright, K.P., "Acute effects of bright light exposure on cortisol levels", *Journal of Biological Rhythms*, 2010; 25(3), pp.208–216. ncbi.nlm.nih.gov/pmc/articles/PMC3686562/. Accessed 31 Mar. 2019

32 Tähkämö, L., Partonen, T. and Pesonen, A.-K., "Systematic review of light exposure impact on human circadian rhythm", *Chronobiology International*, 2019; 36(2), pp.151–170. ncbi.nlm.nih.gov/pubmed/30311830

33 Neal, D.T., Wood, W., Wu, M. and Kurlander, D., "The pull of the past", *Personality and Social Psychology Bulletin*, 2011; 37(11), pp.1428–1437

34 Liu, Y.-Z., Wang, Y.-X. and Jiang, C.-L., "Inflammation: The common pathway of stress-related diseases", *Frontiers in Human Neuroscience*, 2017; 11(16). dx.doi.org/10.3389%2Ffnhum.2017.00316

35 Ghezzi, P., "Role of glutathione in immunity and inflammation in the lung", *International Journal of General Medicine*, 2011; 4, p.105

36 Minich, D.M. and Brown, B.I., "A review of dietary (phyto)nutrients for glutathione support", *Nutrients*, 2019; 11(9), p.2073

37 Palmery, M., Saraceno, A., Vaiarelli, A. and Carlomagno, G., "Oral contraceptives and changes in nutritional requirements", *European Review for Medical and Pharmacological Sciences*, 2013; 17(13), pp.1804–1813. pubmed.ncbi.nlm.nih.gov/23852908/

38 Adlercreutz, H., Pulkkinen, M.O., Hämäläinen, E.K. and Korpela, J.T., "Studies on the role of intestinal bacteria in metabolism of synthetic and

natural steroid hormones", *Journal of Steroid Biochemistry*, 1984; 20(1), pp.217–229

39 Phylactou, M., Clarke, S.A., Patel, B., Baggaley, C., Jayasena, C.N., Kelsey, T.W., Comninos, A.N., Dhillo, W.S. and Abbara, A., "Clinical and biochemical discriminants between functional hypothalamic amenorrhoea (FHA) and polycystic ovary syndrome (PCOS)", *Clinical Endocrinology*, 2010; 95(2)

40 Meczekalski, B., Katulski, K., Czyzyk, A., Podfigurna-Stopa, A. and Maciejewska-Jeske, M., "Functional hypothalamic amenorrhea and its influence on women's health", *Journal of Endocrinological Investigation*, 2014; 37(11), pp.1049–1056

41 Roberts, R.E., Farahani, L., Webber, L. and Jayasena, C., "Current understanding of hypothalamic amenorrhoea", *Therapeutic Advances in Endocrinology and Metabolism*, 2020; 11, p.204201882094585

42 Miller, K.K., Parulekar, M.S., Schoenfeld, E., Anderson, E., Hubbard, J., Klibanski, A. and Grinspoon, S.K., "Decreased leptin levels in normal weight women with hypothalamic amenorrhea: The effects of body composition and nutritional intake", *Journal of Clinical Endocrinology & Metabolism*, 1998; 83(7), pp.2309–2312

43 Pauli, S.A. and Berga, S.L., "Athletic amenorrhea: Energy deficit or psychogenic challenge?", *Annals of the New York Academy of Sciences*, 2010; 1205(1), pp.33–38

44 BEAT: beateatingdisorders.org.uk

45 NEDA: nationaleatingdisorders.org

46 BACP: bacp.org.uk

47 American Counselling Association: counseling.org

48 Rinaldi, N.J., *No Period. Now What? A Guide To Regaining Your Cycles and Improving Your Fertility*, Antica Press Llc, 2019, p.95

Chapter 11

1 Bull, J.R., Rowland, S.P., Scherwitzl, E.B., Scherwitzl, R., Danielsson, K.G. and Harper, J., "Real-world menstrual cycle characteristics of more than 600,000 menstrual cycles", *npj Digital Medicine*, 2019; 2(1), p.4

Index

Note: page numbers in **bold** refer to diagrams; page numbers in *italics* refer to information contained within tables.